THE MIND-BODY MELT

UNLOCK YOUR TRUE POTENTIAL THROUGH FITNESS, MEDITATIONS AND AFFIRMATIONS

DAN EDELSTON & ROB HOWITT

This book is for informational purposes only. It is not intended to serve as a substitute for professional medical advice. The authors and publisher specifically disclaim any and all liability arising directly or indirectly from the use of any information contained in this book. A health care professional should be consulted regarding your specific medical situation. Any product mentioned in this book does not imply endorsement of that product by the author or publisher.

CONTENTS

PREFACE

"All that we are is the result of all that we have thought."

-Buddha

Are you unhappy with the way your body looks?

Do you constantly feel exhausted throughout the day?

Does it seem like your clothes are getting tighter?

Take a moment and consider what your life would be like if every day you looked at yourself in the mirror and thought, "I love how my body looks, I feel fantastic!" We've all had a few moments like this in our lives; it may have been that outfit you purchased for a wedding or that perfectly fitted shirt you tried on in a store. It could have been the way you felt after a new haircut or that moment when someone gave you a sincere compliment. For most of us, these moments are few and far between, and when they do happen, those positive feelings and thoughts of self-worth are fleeting.

Depending on where you are in your life, it might be rather difficult to consider the possibility of waking up every single day and smiling with confidence knowing that you look and feel your best. The idea might even seem like a far off fantasy that is simply too good to be true. But consider what your life would be like if every single day you looked in the mirror and saw a person who was in incredible shape and felt like they could take on the world.

How would your life look? How would you feel about yourself? What would you do with this confidence? How would you act around your family and friends? Who would you talk to that you were previously nervous to approach? What challenges would you take on? Most importantly, what would stop you from accomplishing your every hope and dream?

Don't worry if you're having trouble picturing this new you just yet. It might be tough to visualize the very best version of yourself right now.

However, we have all had at least a few moments we can recall where we truly felt happy about ourselves. There might have even been a day or two where you walked through the world with high levels of self-confidence and radiant self-esteem, the kinds of days where your feelings of inner happiness manifested on the outside. Usually, this happens after going to the gym, having a good workout, or even after a long walk. The beads of sweat on the back of your neck create a sense of calmness and pride which allow you to feel good about yourself. Who knows, maybe you even looked in the mirror and said something nice about yourself!

On days like these, you might have been surrounded by family and friends, and everything just seemed to be right. You were happy, they were happy, and you might have even laughed so hard your stomach hurt. You've taken this feeling of confidence out into the world, and even the cashier at the local grocery store gave you a smile because you brought such a positive energy and light into the world. Later, you put on your favorite music, felt the beat deep within your soul, and experienced a feeling of peace from head to toe.

On this day, you walked through the world with ease. You looked around at others and thought, "Why are they so down? Today is a great day!" You continued to walk around feeling fantastic with a strong sense of purpose, knowing that nothing can bring you down.

"Everyday day should feel this amazing," you think to yourself!

Believe us, it can!

However, this feeling can quickly disappear if you get up the next morning and go through your whole day without any physical activity, without feeling a sense of calmness and without positive words of encouragement you will stumble through the challenges of life rather than walking over them with ease. Your breathing will be shallow and tense. Even worse, with all this stress you will look in the mirror and feel "so-so" or insecure about yourself. The downward spiral will begin; you become critical and self-loathing and will then find something wrong with yourself.

"I want to FEEL as amazing as I did yesterday," you think to yourself, as you stare off into space while the ticks of the clock continue to fade into the background. By the time bedtime arrives, you're burnt out physically, emotionally and mentally. Your day was full of headaches and the littlest of things set you off. You can't quite understand why on one day you felt unstoppable and the next day, so... blah. We've all been there, believe us, it's frustrating beyond belief.

So what do we do? What is the secret to living a life with more confidence? What are the steps you can take to become a better version of yourself? What can you do to look in the mirror every single day and feel your best?

The answer to these questions and the difference between feeling fantastic versus not so great comes down to this:

"Having the courage to take action every day in your life."

Essentially, it all comes down to following a proven system of success which includes molding your body, relaxing the mind and learning how to harmonize the two with your breath. If these concepts sound new or intimidating, don't worry. As you continue reading, you will soon discover the simple and life changing action steps you can take to become the best version of yourself.

This book was inspired and created with years of personal training, meditation, and self-development experience. We took these concepts and created what we call *The Mind Body Melt*. This system is firmly grounded in the idea that you can change your life for the better by taking simple action steps every day to harmonize your mind and body.

Something deep inside inspired you to purchase this book because you know in your heart that you deserve and are capable of more in life. By following this system and adopting new mindsets, you will lose weight, tone muscles, and will look and feel your absolute best in front of a mirror. But more importantly will be the growth that cannot be seen or measured by the eye. *The Mind Body Melt* will instill in you a sense of confidence and self-assurance that is utterly boundless.

With 10+ years of combined personal training experience, we have seen the difficulty our clients have had losing weight, toning muscle and just plain feeling good. As soon as they are close to achieving their goals, some form of a success barrier holds them back.

So what does it take to discover, or rather, become the best version of ourselves?

As the famous Buddha says, "All we are is a result of all we have thought." It all starts with finding the courage to take on new mindsets and change the way we think and feel about ourselves. By following the action steps outlined in this book, you too will be able to change your mindset for the better. And in the process, you will also mold a lean and toned body.

For far too long our minds have imprisoned us; prevented us from evolving and held us back from becoming our ideal selves, both physically and mentally. But just like we have the power to hold ourselves back, we also have the ability to move forward and to set a new course for the ship we call our lives. You DO have the power to control the way you look and the way you feel about yourself. Rest assured this book was created to empower you and help you through this rewarding and worthwhile journey. As long as you follow the steps and believe in your power, your life can change for the better.

We are so excited for the new you.

Here's your beautiful new mind and body,

Dan and Rob

INTRODUCTION

"Nothing is permanent. Everything is subject to change. Being is always becoming."

-Buddha

The simple, yet powerful words of Siddhartha Gautama, more commonly known as Buddha, have been around since the 1st century B.C. They have just as much if not more meaning today as they did over 2,500 years ago. Simply put, we can describe Buddha as the "awakened one." People tend to think of him as someone who was enlightened, or in more basic terms we like to say a person who "just got it."

In our opinion, we feel that Buddha's words cause us to go within, allowing us the opportunity to contemplate the meaning of life. Once inside, we can become aware of things we might have overlooked, put off for another time, or just haven't given deep thought. It's especially true for those of us who do not look and feel the way we want to. As such, we begin to realize why we have not achieved or maintained our dream bodies and start to see what self-defeating behaviors have held us back. More importantly, we discover the reasons why we aren't as happy as we should be.

The centuries old wisdom of Buddha teaches us that all of our problems lie *within* ourselves, not on the outside. Knowing this truth allows us to take back control of our lives. This realization proves we dictate our happiness as well as how we respond to situations. It allows us that sense of independence and autonomy we so desperately crave.

Buddha believed the key to happiness begins with understanding our suffering. Our suffering is the root of unhappiness. It's the reason we are overweight, out of shape and lacking self-confidence. Something deep within is holding us back from the person we want to and can be.

The earliest known teachings of Buddha say, "All we are is the result of all we have thought." Simply put, if we believe we are out of shape, overweight, and think poorly about ourselves, we have created a sense of reality which is congruent to this belief. These feelings will continue to feed and perpetuate the never-ending cycle of negative self-worth.

Within this book, you will discover the life-changing system that will not only get you in fantastic shape but will help you relax and harmonize your mind and body connection. Through *The Mind Body Melt*, you will learn what you can do in your life to become the happy and confident person you not only want to be, but deserve to be.

By applying our simple principles, you will put into motion a new way of thinking, a new way of taking action, and a new way of being. You'll soon find yourself inspired to work out! Your mind will change from thinking, "I have to work out" to "I "want to work out!"

Our system is grounded in what we call the 3 S's: Shaping, Shifting, and Strengthening.

It looks a little something like this:

*Shape the body

*Shift racing thoughts

*Strengthen the mind-body connection.

The three S's are nothing new. You probably already know someone who is shaping their body into ideal form through exercise. Some people are shifting their racing thoughts through meditation, while others are strengthening their mind-body connection in various ways.

However, these individuals are not following a proven formula for success. They are missing out on a system that creates long lasting results and sustained motivation, a method that would challenge them mentally and physically like never before.

Rest assured, by following *The Mind Body Melt* you will begin to look and feel your best through concrete action steps which have been tested and proven successful on ourselves as well as our clients.

Regardless of what has happened to you in the past, everything can change for the better starting right now. Whether you are a man or woman, young or old, busy beyond belief or bored out of your mind, this system will work for you. Even better, you can do it any time of the day. It's totally up to you!

By taking action, you will soon realize how much more life has to offer. Your newly increased, deep-rooted self-confidence will open new doors and opportunities right before your very eyes. You'll find yourself happier more often and, of course, you will find yourself fitting into clothes you haven't worn in years.

Even better, you'll become an inspiration for others in-cluding your family and friends. People will notice your improved physical appearance and will feel your hap-piness and energy radiating everywhere you go. The feeling will become contagious, and they'll ask you "what is your secret?" Feel free to share this book with everyone you know. Heck, even give them your copy for free because that's what this is all about; we are here to empower, to improve, and to make people's lives bet-ter.

There's just one thing…

If you are going to become the best version of yourself and plan on achieving all of these beautiful things you are starting to envision, you have to be willing to take action. Just reading this book alone will not turn you into the person you want to become. Don't be one of those individuals who read countless self-development books, posts quotes about positivity all over Facebook, and attends endless seminars only to forget all about taking any actual action. Too many people get excited about the possibility of doing something big and then rationalize that as being enough action. Don't be this average, everyday person who settles for life as it passes them by; instead become the person who takes action, begins to think differently, and finds a purpose and meaning to their story.

Don't worry about past experiences where you tried to step up and did not get what you wanted. Everything in life, good or bad, is a learning experience. We always tell ourselves, "We don't fail, we learn." You can't know more about yourself and what life has to offer if you don't step outside of your comfort zone.

We just have to find the courage and the confidence to take that first step beyond the walls we have built for ourselves. This might sound scary but fear not, we are here to guide you every step of the way.

As you continue reading this book, you will learn the exact system we have put in place to change your life for the better. The system is easy to follow and is very user-friendly. However, before we delve in, there is a concept you must first understand. The following is imperative to your success, and unless you embody it now, you will not achieve your highest physical, mental, and emotional goals.

Understand this,

You will only obtain your dream body and maintain higher levels of happiness if you begin to feel good today.

This concept might sound a bit strange, especially to those of you who are currently unhappy with your bodies. You might think, well how can I feel good if I don't look good right now? If I am seeking my dream body, but I'm already happy now, why would I even work for it?

It is quite a paradox indeed but stay with us because you will soon see how the importance of feeling good now can change your life moving forward.

When it comes to fitness goals, most people give up before they see any progress. The biggest problem comes from seeing exercise as a chore, something difficult that "has to be done." Then, we associate the FEELING of "having to workout" as a negative one, and the pursuit of a healthier and leaner body ceases to exist.

Even worse, the idea of achieving an ideal body falls short for many individuals because they feel deep within that they are simply not enough. For example, they might feel they don't deserve to have their dream body because some form of a success barrier is holding them back. It could be they heard the words: too fat, too skinny, too this, too that. Or maybe they felt self-conscious about a particular part of their body or worried what others would be thinking about them. Whatever it may have been, the result was always the same. The feeling of not being worthy or not being enough continues to perpetuate. It's then given power and the dream of achieving a fitness goal disappears before it ever even started.

Could it get any worse?

Yes, it can!

Especially, when it comes to looking at ourselves in the mirror, our negative thoughts are the biggest self-defeating barrier of all time. Whether we are getting dressed, brushing our teeth, or taking a glance in a reflecting window, our thoughts are always highly critical. "I need to lose weight," "I need to tone my muscles," "I need to flatten my stomach." No matter what we may look like, we find fault trying to live up to what we think society's standards want us to be. We believe, "When I lose this amount of weight, or get a flat stomach or have some definition in my muscles, *then* I'll be happy. When that happens, *then* I'll be the person I want to be." It's an endless cycle of chasing the future happier version of you.

It doesn't have to be this way...

Find the courage and strength that you have buried deep within. Find that little light of confidence that has dimmed throughout the years. Find that inner spark that makes you feel worthy and powerful. Grab a hold. Harness it. Use it. Make a choice to change the way you feel today.

By changing how you feel today, you can minimize these negative thoughts. By limiting these self-defeating thoughts, you begin to feel better about yourself. By feeling better about yourself, you start to treat yourself better. By treating yourself better, you take the necessary actions to perpetuate these feelings, i.e. exercising, and meditating. By exercising, you begin to shape your body toward your more ideal image. By meditating after exercise, you allow your mind to relax, and by using affirmations, you reinforce this new you. Before long you look in the mirror and have positive thoughts that result in feeling good inside and out. By utilizing this approach, you have completely transformed the cycle from one of negative self-criticism to one of positive self-empowerment.

Now you are beginning to see what we mean.

Remember…

You will only obtain your dream body and maintain higher levels of happiness if you start to feel good today.

So how do we get there?

What will it take to get there?

It all starts by working on the 3S's:

*Shape the body

*Shift racing thoughts

*Strengthen the mind-body connection.

The Mind Body Melt empowers you to finally take the necessary action to change your life for the better. When you apply the 3 S's, you take the first step on this very rewarding journey to becoming the best version of yourself. Instead of taking a shortcut or finding an easy way to make yourself look and feel better, you are taking action and embodying the person you want to become.

We know this from personal experience; we've spent years upon years researching and experimenting with various methods to find a formula to enable people to look and feel their best. It's been a long journey of experimentation, self-growth, and self-empowerment. In this book, we've compiled everything we have learned and used to help ourselves and countless others find success.

And who are we?

We are Dan Edelston and Rob Howitt.

But first, let's start with the primary author, me, Dan.

I am a certified personal trainer, hold a master's degree in Rehabilitation Counseling, am a certified Reiki Master, have been meditating for 10+ years, and have read hundreds of self-development books in all areas of personal growth.

After assisting clients in reaching their goals of losing weight and toning their bodies, I saw some pretty amazing results. However, the outcomes were not long lasting. My clients would achieve these great bodies for a few weeks only to a few months later sabotage themselves by putting the weight back on and then some. It's as if their physical body changed, but their mind still lacked confidence, self-esteem, and happiness. It was frustrating to see so many people get to where they wanted to be, only to have it taken away by none other than themselves. I knew something had to change; there had to be a way to maintain these results.

As I began developing training programs for my clients, I turned to my mentor trainer and fellow co-author, Rob Howitt, who showed me even more efficient ways to put together exercise programs. He taught me how High-Intensity Interval Training (HIIT) is the most efficient way for clients to lose weight and tone muscles in less than 30 minutes per workout.

One day I told Rob about my problem with helping my clients sustain results and surprisingly, he said he had the same issue with his clients. Then, a few days later we were talking, and it became evident we were both having a stressful day. We decided to do a 20-minute workout together in hopes that maybe we would feel a little relief. The workout was quite intense using the ever challenging HIIT training. Afterward, he reported that he felt better physically but was still upset about a few things he could not get off his mind

Can you relate?

Some personal trainers will tell you that if you work out, you will feel much better afterward. It's true to some extent; we do feel better post-workout, but are we able to let go of our mental and emotional problems? And for how long do we feel good? How long is the great feeling sustained after a vigorous training session?

It was at this moment on what seemed like an ordinary day back in 2010, that I decided to try something different. Something that would completely change the way I trained my clients and thought about the impact of fitness on both the body and the mind.

A few months prior I had talked to Rob about the benefits of meditation which he had politely listened to but thought to be nothing more than new-age nonsense. He had tried it a few times himself but felt he never had success. Since he was in a little bit of a better mood this day, I decided to see if he wanted to give meditation a try. He said, "Why the hell not, I'll try anything at this point."

My suggestion at this time was two-fold; I brought up this idea because during this time I was on a break from meditating. It had been a few months since I took the time and effort to meditate and I could feel myself becoming antsier and stressed out about little, unimportant things.

We were both ready to give it a try, so to begin, I had Rob sit in the lotus position and took him through a brief 5-minute meditation to help him let go of the uneasiness in his mind. We performed a powerful technique that you will learn later in this book. During the meditation, Rob not only became aware of his problems but was able to let them go. He didn't suppress them; he truly let go.

At the end of the meditation, Rob slowly opened his eyes and looked over at me with an entirely peaceful demeanor. His eyes were bright, his shoulders were relaxed, and he had a satisfied and sincere smile on his face. He told me he had not felt this relaxed in decades!

Rob felt we might be on to something. He had tried to meditate before but was never successful, yet something about this time was different. Because Rob exercised first, his mind wasn't racing, and he was able to focus on his breathing and listen to the words as I guided him through the meditation.

It was at this moment where I realized that this same technique might also work with my clients. Soon, I began having them meditate after their workouts. I even tried it on myself, and I have to tell you the results were utterly profound! My clients began reporting they were happier, felt better about their bodies when they looked in the mirror and had a calmer and clearer mindset as they went about their day.

These individuals continued to lose weight, tone their bodies and felt better about the way they looked. However, there was still something missing. Their results seemed to last longer, meaning they kept the weight off and maintained their strength and muscle tone. But after a few months, they would fall back into their self-defeating behaviors and the success barriers would again persist.

As you will see in the following chapters, there is one more key ingredient about *The Mind Body Melt,* which will deepen and strengthen the mind-body connection. It's something you may have heard of before; however, it needs to be performed at the exact right moment if you are going to re-program your subconscious mind. Otherwise, you are wasting your time.

The purpose of sharing these stories isn't to brag; instead, we are looking to bring hope and inspiration to your life. We want to show you that no matter what has held you back in the past, you can start again and make a change. We've seen the most challenging and stubborn clients transform their lives by following our principles. We know you can do it too!

The difference is walking the walk. We wouldn't have the guts to go for our dreams and write this book if it wasn't for following our rules and seeing firsthand how to harmonize the mind-body connection and build a self-empowerment state of mind.

We learned everything through years of education, personal experience, and endless fitness experimentation with ourselves and with our clients. We have seen countless individuals put the work into losing weight only to gain it all back. And we can both share with you that nothing is more devastating to a trainer to see that happen.

Along with this journey, we've managed to help countless people transform their lives by using this unique system. We've seen people rise from the ashes of yesterday like a Phoenix being reborn for a greater purpose. We've had the honor and privilege of witnessing our clients as they grew wings, took flight, and became the person they have always wanted to be.

But we aren't perfect by any means; the journey to finding even more efficient ways to harmonize the mind and body and more methods to look and feel your best is a never ending process. However, what we do know is that this formula works.

This book is a summary of and the results of years and years of self-development, experimentation, and countless personal training experience. As with any great discovery, we wish we had come across this formula sooner, but we are so thankful that we can share it with you now.

If you are like us, you know that you DESERVE more. You deserve to look and feel your best. You deserve everything life has to offer. Don't let another day of feeling bad about yourself and not looking your best continue. It's time to put yourself back in the driver seat of your life, and get on the road to a better you!

PART I

FITNESS

O

Chapter 1

OUR BIGGEST PROBLEM

The number one complaint we get with any new clients is, "I want to lose weight."

Think about it, how many times have you thought, "I'm too heavy, I need to lose weight, I can't fit into my clothes, ugh, I don't like the way I look, I went up a size, I have never been this heavy." No matter what we are thinking, we never seem to run out of these awful thoughts and feelings.

Thoughts about our weight are ever present; whether looking at the calories on the side of a cereal box, standing on a scale in our doctor's office or noticing an overweight person standing in line at a fast food restaurant. Our minds are almost always thinking about how much we weigh on a daily basis, whether we'd like to admit it or not. And for some, it's all consuming.

Ideally, we want to have healthy, lean, fit bodies. We want to be that certain jean size, we want to say we are our ideal weight, and we absolutely want to love the way we look.

So how do we get there?

To achieve our ideal body weight, we need to address the 3 Keys to Weight Loss which include: Intensity, Creating Your Ideal Workout and learning about Weight Loss Tips that really work.

Chapter 2

HOW TO INCREASE YOUR INTENSITY

Are you truly pushing yourself? Are you really giving it all you've got?

After training hundreds of clients, it has become clear that many people are not giving their all during exercise. Now, we are not saying to push yourself to the point of injury or passing out, but you must understand this:

"Your body can do a lot more than you think it can."

You can exert more during your workouts and, if you do, the results will be monumental.

This might be news to you, but ideally, your workouts should be no longer than a total of 45 minutes.

I can already hear you saying, "Aren't longer workouts better?"

No, they are not. There have been numerous studies to prove otherwise, in fact, 30-45 minutes are ideal. Let's take a look. We promise not to bore you either.

According to the American Journal of Physiology, 30 minutes of daily training provides equally effective weight loss as a 60-minute workout.[1]

Additionally, the World Health Organization recommends between 30-45 minutes of exercise for the ideal duration of fitness.[2]

Not to get all scientific and put you to sleep, but if you perform a Google search for Cortisol and working out for more than 2 hours. You will learn that working out for this amount of time, even at moderate levels, causes your body to release this stress hormone which in turn causes your body to store fat and water.[3]

"Well that can't be good" you must be thinking, and you're correct! You begin to store fat because your body thinks it's in survival mode, holding onto everything you ingest for fear there might not be enough food later.

Now that we know this information, the question becomes, how do we monitor our intensity during this ideal 30-45-minute period?

The answer is quite simple, it all comes down to how we feel, and scientifically, how we can elevate our heart rate.

With exercise, the intensity is subjective; meaning what you believe to be a high level of effort might be low for another person.

To get a better sense of how much intensity we need to be exerting we need to understand the difference between moderate versus vigorous levels of exercise.

At a moderate level, you might feel your breath is getting heavier, but you aren't fatigued. After several minutes, you could begin to feel some warmth and perspiration emanating from your skin. At this point, you can still carry on a conversation without gasping for air. Whether you are talking about how you can't believe your friend did "that" or how much you hate working out, you can still convey your message.

However, with vigorous exercise, your breath becomes shallow and quick. Sweat is pouring out after only a few minutes of exertion. Additionally, you can barely say more than a few words without having to pause for breath.

Keep in mind the last thing you ever want to do is push yourself to the point where you get light headed and feel like you're going to pass out.

But, honestly ask yourself, "Am I getting to a vigorous level of intensity at any point in my work out?" Your workout should not focus on sustaining a maximum heart rate, but you should question if the workout has elevated your heart rate at any given point and time during your training session.

7

*Note: Be sure to speak with a healthcare professional before starting any exercise program.)

If you are having a difficult time trying to comprehend how hard to exercise, we do have the formula to make this concept easier to understand.

We are going to get a little scientific but stay with us; we won't overwhelm you.

Ideally, we like to see our clients measure their heart rate. Your heart rate tells you how many times your heart beats per minute. To get our ideal numbers, we calculate our Maximum Heart Rate which is 220 minus your age.[4]

(220-Your Age= Your Maximum Heart Rate)

For example, if you are 35 years old, your maximum heart rate would be 185. (220-35=185).

Be sure to calculate your maximum heart rate (220-age).

Now that we have the information, we want to see where we are performing moderate and vigorous levels of exercise intensity.

We only have two more calculations to perform. Believe us we do not want to make this book about math and equations. They are not our strong points and put most people to sleep. However, the importance of knowing these numbers is essential to your weight loss. So let's take a look at your numbers.

According to the Centers for Disease Control and Prevention (CDC):

Moderate Exercise is 50-70% of your max HR[4]

Vigorous Exercise is 70-85% of max HR[4] (Target Zone - this is where you burn the most calories)

*Note we recommend if you are new to exercise stay to the lower numbers 50% moderate and 70% vigorous.

Hold on because now we need a calculator…But don't worry we will guide you through, it's quite simple. Remember, these numbers are significant.

For simplicity purposes, calculate the following:

Moderate Exercise- (Your Max heart rate multiplied by .5 and then by .7)

For example, our 35-year-old would have an ideal moderate metabolic rate between 92.5 (185 x. 5) and 129.5 (185 x .7).

Knowing this information allows us to realize that if this individual's heart rate is between 92.5 and 129.5, they are performing a moderate exercise. However, they are not burning the ideal amount of calories to lose weight.

To find out what we need to do to burn those calories we need to find our ideal heart rate for vigorous exercise.

Vigorous Exercise- (Your Max heart rate multiplied by .7 and then by .85)

The 35-year-old would have a target heart rate range between 129.5 (185 x.7 and 157.25 (185 x .85).

Now that you have your numbers you know exactly where you need to be to burn the ideal amount of calories.

But how long should I stay in these heart rate zones?

Depending on the type of workout you perform, your amount of time in these ranges will vary. Even with brisk walking or jogging, you can burn calories. One thing to realize is that if you aren't getting to your vigorous heart rate zone for at least a few seconds to a few minutes, you are not adequately maximizing your calorie burning potential. Believe us, we've seen many people go to the gym, only to slowly pedal on a bike or mindlessly spend an hour on an elliptical without ever spending one second in the vigorous heart rate zone.

Don't be this person!

If you want to burn the most calories while spending the majority of your workout in the vigorous zone for the shortest amount of time, you need to try HIIT.

HIIT TRAINING

High-Intensity Interval Training or HIIT is a form of exercise which switches between short periods of anaerobic exercise with less-intense recovery periods.[5] With this style of training, you will burn more calories and fat in a shorter period. Better yet, it creates something called an after burn which means you are burning calories even after you have finished your workout.[6]

Yes, you can burn calories while you are sitting or sleeping for a period after your workout.

Research has shown this effect can last for 24-72 hours after fairly intense exercise; it's called the "After Burn" effect or EPOC which stands for Excessive Post-Exercise Oxygen Consumption.[7]

Simply put, the After Burn takes place because the more intense your workout, the more oxygen you consume after your workout which keeps your heart rate elevated; because your energy expenditure after your workout remains high, calories continue to burn.

In HIIT your goal is to workout at 85% of your target. As you can imagine, there are many types of programs out there which vary regarding their exercises and amount of time.

If we are creating a workout for beginners, the routine might look like this:

6 exercise movements each performed for 30 seconds followed by a 30 second period of rest for a total of 2 to 3 rounds.

If we are creating a workout for clients at intermediate levels, the routine might look like this:

6 exercise movements each performed for 40 seconds followed by a 20 second period of rest for a total of 3 to 4 rounds.

And for those advanced individuals, the routine would like something like this:

6 exercise movements each performed for 50 seconds followed by a 10 second period of rest for a total of 3 to 4 rounds.

Keep in mind; everyone is completely different regarding their exercise goals and levels of experience.

If you are interested in discovering the ideal routine for yourself, we highly recommend that you check out our YouTube channel called *The Mind-Body Melt* or hop on over to our website: www.TheMind-BodyMelt.com. It's a great place to start, especially if you are new to exercise or are looking for a new kind of workout.

Right now you're probably thinking and beginning to understand that you need to add more intensity to your current exercise program. You might also be thinking, "What else can I do to get my dream body?" "I've been told exercise is only a part of weight loss?"

Keep in mind, exercise is a weight loss accelerator; it can help you lose those stubborn pounds quickly through burning calories. It's also an excellent way to remain strong and flexible. However, the biggest key to weight loss comes down to nutrition.

Chapter 3

HOW TO CHANGE YOUR EATING HABITS

For many, the word diet provokes thoughts of anxiety, confusion, and frustration. It's a concept that people stress over and can never seem to grasp how to implement the right eating in their lives properly.

Can you relate?

You may have tried countless diet programs to lose weight, only to gain it back a few months later. You've gone out and bought the healthiest foods, only to have them sit in the fridge and go bad because you didn't have time to prepare your meals or became bored with eating the same foods over and over again. You might have even stayed with this diet program for up to a full year, but where are you now?

Unlike most books which delve into the depths of nutrition, we want to keep it simple and focus on basic healthy eating. We don't want to overwhelm you, make your head spin, or give you overwhelming anxiety every time you have a meal.

We've broken down the exact tips we've used with our clients to assist and coach them on their weight loss journey. Some of these concepts might be familiar to you, and you may have heard them hundreds of times. Even so, try your absolute best to absorb the material instead of just skimming over concepts you have seen before. Try to apply these tips instead of saying, "I already know that." It's one thing to know something; it's another to implement it and make it a habit. The key to conquering nutrition is to make it a habit!

Over the years thousands and thousands of books have been written on what to eat, each one claiming to be more powerful and effective than the next. There is no doubt each one provides at least one nugget of useful information and helpful weight loss tips. We encourage you to read some of these books if you want to gain a deeper understanding of dieting and to compare and contrast different methodologies.

While useful, the amount of information presented in these books can feel overwhelming and difficult to grasp. Due to the inability to understand the material, we've seen some individuals attempt to combine the information from different books where they bounce back from one diet to another. Others will stick to a diet for a few weeks only to give up because they don't see results.

The main problem here is the word "diet" because a diet is temporary, restricting and usually doesn't last too long. A person on a diet knows there is an end in sight and as a result, only eats specific foods for a certain amount of days, weeks or months.

As a result, we need to change the way our mind thinks about the foods we eat. We want healthy eating to become a sustained habit, something you easily do for years if not the rest of your life; which is why we need to clear up any confusion regarding the concept of dieting and nutrition. We do not plan on giving you complex information, 20 ingredient recipes, or a list of foods to avoid. Instead, we will discuss the power of habits.

Most of our daily habits are automatic. We don't necessarily know why many of our everyday actions occur, but we keep doing them, and they persist almost unconsciously. Whether it's eating that unhealthy on the go breakfast burrito, that candy bar at lunch, that late night bowl of ice cream, or buying that bag of chips while grocery shopping, we aren't consciously thinking about what we are doing. Instead, we are subconsciously sabotaging ourselves at the expense of our bodies.

Over the years, we've provided our clients with a few simple, yet powerful tips to help them lose weight and change their bad habits and are now happy to pass on this knowledge and share these secrets of success with you. Keep in mind some of these may sound familiar, but the real goal is not only to reinforce these concepts but to take action.

Chapter 4

WEIGHT LOSS TIPS THAT WORK

The first tip occurs at the one location we have the most control over yet let our impulses and drives stop us from making the right choices. The first habit we need to start working on immediately is to make better choices of the foods we buy in the supermarket.

If you think about it, you are stocking your household inventory. You have control over what foods go in your refrigerator and your kitchen cabinets. You have the influence of what you or your family eats. And you have the power to make the necessary change. With that, our best piece of advice is to, shop the perimeter of the supermarket.

Yes, some supermarkets have their bakery and frozen foods sections strategically placed around the perimeter. But let's look at the real message we are trying to convey.

What is on the perimeter of grocery stores?

Typically, this is where you will find your produce section, your meat section, and your fish counter. By spending the majority of your time if not all your time in these areas only, you will avoid the cookies, the potato chips, and most importantly, you will avoid the chemically rich foods located in each and every aisle.

What about dairy?

Yes, Greek yogurt or cottage cheese could be in your nutrition plan, but if you are looking to avoid gaining weight and making those poor food choices, keep it simple: Fruits, Vegetables, Meats and Fish.

Also, while in the supermarket be sure to avoid almost anything that comes in a box or a bag. Most of the time, these products will have an overwhelming amount of sugar, fat, or chemicals. Stay away at all cost, especially if the ingredients are words you can't even pronounce. If you can't avoid these items, try to replace them with something that is a 100% fruit juice, 100% whole-grains, etc.

These are simple changes that you can make during your short trip to the grocery store. But what can you do at home? What happens once the foods packed away and the pantries fully stocked with all of those healthier options? What about when that chocolate craving hits after dinner?

As many of us know the foods we eat at home are another culprit to our weight gain. We eat more than we should, and it's always at the worst possible hours.

Throughout the day our willpower diminishes, so by the evening, our ability to say no to these tasty treats is nearly impossible. To avoid falling into this common pitfall, we encourage you to take the "Plate Approach."

What is the Plate Approach you might ask?

If weight loss is what you are striving for, try this,

Divide your plate into three sections; 50% vegetables, 25% protein and 25% carbohydrates.

The healthy carbs you can eat are sweet potatoes, rice, and quinoa. If you're still finding it difficult to lose weight avoid the carbs and make it 50% protein and 50% vegetables

What about fruit? Can I eat fruit?

Yes, and No...

Eating fruit can be beneficial due to their many nutrients including vitamins and minerals. However, the timing of when to eat these foods is essential. When we eat fruit in the morning or afternoon it provides us with the healthy benefits we need such as essential nutrients and fiber.[8] As we go through the day, the sugar is burned off and not stored as fat.

However, when we eat fruit at night, the sugar is not burnt off because we are not active or exercising. The sugar then gets stored as fat and causes you to gain weight!

Have you said this before, "But I'm eating healthy, I eat fruit, why can't I lose weight?"

Eat your fruit, but eat it wisely.

Notably, last simple tip to losing weight involves something we all need and have on a daily basis.

It's something so simple to understand, yet most of us don't get enough of it.

Do you think you know what it is…?"

It's water.

Water you say?

How the bleeping hell is water going to help me lose weight?

Before you throw your arms in the air and give up, let's take a closer look…

The Importance of Water

Over the years, numerous studies have examined how water can aid in weight loss.

These research studies concluded the following:

• Drinking water increases the number of calories your burn.[9]

• A study of overweight women found that after drinking 34 oz. of water per day for 12 months, these women on average lost an extra 4.4 pounds.[10]

• Drinking water before breakfast reduced the amount of calories consumed during the meal.[11]

• Drinking cold water makes our body burn extra calories to warm up your body temperature.[12]

• People who drink water on average consume 200 fewer calories per day because it is calorie free.[13]

So there you have it.

By beginning to make simple changes, we can lose weight and keep it off. Weight loss shouldn't be a stressful, aggravating, or time-consuming experience. All you have to do is eat smarter, drink water, don't over-think it, and apply the habits. We promise you will see a dramatic difference.

However, before we can address the mental component of this book, there is one more area we need to address. It involves the consistency of our exercise. We've already discussed the importance HIIT and what to eat, yet there is still something missing on your weight loss journey.

The final pillar of weight loss is consistency, meaning, how often a person exercises.

Typical questions include:

How many days should I work out? How long of a workout do I need? What kind of exercises should I do?

Chapter 5

YOUR IDEAL WORKOUT

First, you must understand that everyone's goals are different and without sitting down with you and creating a customized weight loss plan, it is not an easy answer. However, there are some good foundational principles you can follow to ensure your motivation stays high, and you attain your goals.

After seeing hundreds of gym members give up on their goals and burn themselves out, we have found the ideal number of days to get your heart rate pumping and tone your body is between 2-4 days per week.

Now realize we are talking about HIIT. We are not including other great forms of exercise such as walking, yoga, or light jogging. These forms of cardio will take place on your non-HIIT days. (Be sure to check out our 30-day challenge at the end of the book to learn more).

With that, we've found two days to be the minimum requirement to maintain motivation and begin to see a change in your body. If you're working out just one day per week, you are wasting your time.

While two days a week of exercise isn't ideal for long-term success, we feel it is a great place to start for the first month, especially if you are new to fitness or have struggled in the past. For those who love to workout and push themselves, they will find four days to be a better alternative.

By working out for four days per week, you can burn more calories, engage more muscles, develop a greater sense of motivation as well as reinforce new habits. Exercising this many days per week is also beneficial for a person who is naturally full of energy or who already has years of fitness experience.

What about exercising intensely for 5 to 6 days a week?

Personally, we don't recommend intense exercise for that many days per week. The reason being is that we've found when clients push themselves 5 to 6 times a week with intense interval training; they end up burning out and losing motivation. Remember, life is about balance. Perform 2-4 days of intense interval training and then 1-3 days per week of light cardio.

Strive for workouts between 30-45 minutes in total. We've optimized the 30-minute window, so not even one second goes to waste. As long as you are pushing yourself and working hard during those 30 minutes, you are doing enough to burn fat, tone muscle, and increase your cardiovascular output. From our experience, a typical 45-minute workout is just a 30-minute workout that takes too much time. Because we are living such busy lives, it's ideal to make the best use out of our time, especially if we want to spend more time on the important things such as family or work.

Since we are all limited on time yet still want to achieve our fitness goals, the best exercise we have found is HIIT. As previously discussed, HIIT is a form of exercise which switches between short periods of anaerobic exercise with less-intense recovery periods. This kind of training will burn more calories and fat than most workouts out there in less time. Better yet, it creates an after burn which means you are burning calories even after you have finished your workout. Yes, that means you can burn calories while you are sitting or sleeping for a period after your workout.

Now during these workouts, you should incorporate body weight exercises. By using just your body, you give yourself the freedom to perform these exercises at anytime and anywhere. You don't have to buy expensive gym equipment or an endless supply of dumbbells to sculpt your ideal body.

Turn to the next page and take a look at a typical HIIT training session so you can see how to structure your workout.

The Workout

1 Minute Breathing Warmup- *(Sitting in the lotus position breathe in for 6 seconds, hold for 3 seconds, exhale for 3 seconds, hold for 3 seconds.. continue until 1 minute has passed)*

1 Minute Dynamic Warmup- *(Perform squats at a slow pace for 30 seconds followed by arm circles for 30 seconds)*

8 Minute Interval Round- which consists of four strength training exercises. 40 Seconds on 20 Seconds off for 8 minutes. (Pushups, Squats, Mountain Climbers and Glut e Bridges).

1 Minute Rest

8 Minute Interval Round- which consists of 4 exercises. 40 Seconds on 20 Seconds rest for 8 minutes. (Jumping Jacks, Mountain Climbers, Burpees and Skaters).

Four minute "Finisher Workout."- (Ab Crunches, Low Leg Lift, Side Plank Left Side then Side Plank Right Side). Perform each for 30 seconds straight for (4) minutes).

Be sure to google the exercises that are unfamiliar

With HIIT, you experience the calorie burning effects of cardio combined with the muscle toning of weight training. Why spend time on a treadmill and then lift weights when you could combine the benefits of both into one highly productive workout?

If you would like to experience the life changing results of a specially designed HIIT training program, be sure to check out www.TheMind-BodyMelt.com where you can purchase our six week Mind Body Melt workout.

For those of you looking to save some money and want to start off on your own, be sure to check out our 30-day challenge at the end of this book for a more modified yet still highly effective workout for your mind and body.

PART II

MEDITATIONS

Chapter 6

THE NEED TO MEDITATE AFTER EXERCISE

On the journey to looking and feeling our best, many of us get caught up in the notion of only looking good. We obsess over the numbers on the scale; we look in the mirror with criticism and tell ourselves that one day we will be in fantastic shape.

To make ourselves feel better, we begin exercising and change the ways we eat in an attempt to accomplish our goals. While this is a noble effort, the problem is that we only focus on our aesthetics. We don't make a deep identity level change and instead, keep the same self-defeating thoughts constant in our minds. No matter how skinny or fit we become, we still feel we are not enough.

It's an endless cycle as there always seem to be a problem area on our bodies we want to improve. For some reason, we can't look in the mirror and just be happy with ourselves. Therefore, it is no wonder why so many individuals never FEEL their best or even feel "okay" for that matter.

We knew something had to change, especially after years and years of seeing so many of our personal training clients not feel as good as they looked. Soon we began experimenting with how we could change a person's mindset. Initially, I (Dan) started using techniques I had acquired from my Master Degree in Rehabilitation Counseling. I tried Motivational Interviewing Psychoanalysis, Cognitive-Behavioral-Therapy, Assertive-Communication and even a Positive Belief Record. While these techniques made small improvements in the way my clients thought about themselves, I noticed they still didn't FEEL good about themselves.

That's when I decided to try something that has had a profound life- changing impact not only for me but my clients as well. So much so, that it has inspired me to create the Mind Body Melt and share it with the world. My secret to helping people look and feel their best is simple:

"Meditate after Exercise"

The benefits of meditation are immense, and we will cover those in greater detail. But first, let's discuss how meditation can allow you to finally not only feel amazing but the best you've ever felt.

Many of us have not had success meditating because we cannot calm our minds, turn off our brains, and control our breathing. However, if you perform a meditation after a workout, you're going to notice it's a lot easier to get into that kind of relaxed state.

Why is that?

Typically, when we try to meditate without working out before hand, we are trapped in our heads; our minds are racing, and our thoughts are nonstop. There is also muscular tension in our bodies and excess energy that needs to be released. It's not the ideal combination for meditative success.

However, when we exercise first, we see profound effects take place because we are not in our heads. This change occurs when energy begins to move down to our body enhancing the mind-body connection. Since we are moving at such a rapid rate, our mind can't focus on anything else besides getting us to the next movement. It's is a form of meditation as we are focusing steadily on just one task.

Exercise helps keep our egos in check. It also humbles us, grounds us and brings us back to reality. When we meditate without exercise, we might think about things like "I don't need to meditate, I'm all right," "I don't have time to meditate," or "I can't relax, I have things to do!" By simply sweating and moving we quiet down our egos, lower the stress of our day to day struggles and connect with our true selves. When we are engaged in exercise and push ourselves, our egos will not be able to self-doubt.

Exercise also helps break up the muscular tension our bodies hold from our emotions. Have you ever had butterflies in your stomach or pain in your neck? Typically, these are the internal manifestations of stress. We have a tendency to hold our tension in our neck, causing unnecessary strain and pain. If we are worried or anxious, our stomachs become uneasy and weak.

During a fight or flight situation, we experience a trauma, which is then stored in our body as muscular tension.[14] It could be something as minor as an argument with a loved one, work stressors, family expectations, or any situation where something happens to you, and your body tenses up. As a result, this energy of fear is stored in our body and can manifest as physical problems for years. By exercising, we can release these emotions, and our bodies can finally relax. From there, our chances to meditate greatly increase.

As you can see, there are numerous benefits to meditation, yet so few people attempt to perform this practice. And those that do seem to believe they aren't doing it right.

The question then becomes "How can we learn to meditate and feel our best?"

To answer this question, we need to take a more in-depth look at meditation. We want to give you the tools necessary to perform this life-changing practice so you can finally start feeling your best.

What is Meditation?

A simple Google search will yield endless results in an attempt to define meditation. Personally, we've found with many individuals it can feel overwhelming and confusing to grasp the essence of the practice. However, after years of meditating as well as speaking with and coaching numerous individuals, we've found the best way to describe this practice is:

"A method of relaxing and transforming the mind for the better."

Now at some point in our lives, we start to realize there are many things, circumstances as well as events that we cannot control. It could be anything from a car accident to the wrath of Mother Nature's destruction or even just plain bad luck, and when it occurs it leaves us feeling stuck, overwhelmed and frustrated.

Thankfully, we can change the way our mind handles these situations and gain a sense of control. By taking responsibility for how we respond and reflect, we can alleviate our anxieties, hatred, fears and most importantly, the way we feel about ourselves.

To overcome our typical negative auto responses to external stimuli, we need to go within, reflect, and let go. Meditation encourages us to focus on positive emotions and creates a sense of calming and a connection to nature and one another. It forms in us an ability to develop a deeper focus. The more we practice meditation, the more we experience this profoundly relaxed state of mind. Soon, we begin to love ourselves again and feel a transformation from a negative body image to one of happiness and satisfaction.

The benefits of meditation are so immense that we could write a whole book on only that one particular topic. The practice brings a deep level of self-awareness and a better connection to the world around us. It helps us connect with our true selves and become mindful of what is serving and not serving us.

In combining fitness with meditation, we have seen some life changing results. The key to becoming aware and transcending our mind is to relax and reflect without judgment. By having our clients meditate after their workout, we have seen an increase in their overall happiness, confidence, and a general sense of calmness with the chaotic world around them. They have reported a closer connection with others, increased confidence in social situations, and a better understanding of their life purpose.

Wouldn't you like to feel the same way?

In addition to the benefits we have seen from meditation, there are numerous studies also show the physical, mental, and emotional benefits.

The following is a list of outcomes from a number of studies showing how meditation improves our bodies, mind, and mood.[15]

For our bodies, meditation:

- Lowers blood pressure
- Improves breathing
- Decreases inflammation
- Reduces risk of Alzheimer's
- Helps to manage heart rate
- Increases longevity

For our minds, meditation:
- Improves focus, attention, and ability to work under stress
- Improves information processing and decision-making
- Gives us more resilience toward pain
- Increases capacity to focus even with distractions
- Improves learning, memory, and self-awareness

For our moods, meditation:
- Decreases depression
- Regulates our mood and anxiety
- Reduces stress
- Increases gray matter in the brain
- Reduces symptoms of a panic disorder

These are just a few of the many benefits of this simple practice. Currently, more research is being conducted across the world to see what other kinds of positive life changing benefits can come from the practice of going within.

We are excited to learn more and will be sure to share them with you in upcoming E-Books and YouTube videos.

Misconceptions of Meditation

If you are new to the practice, understand there is a lot of misinformation which leads many to avoid meditation altogether. Typically, it comes from word of mouth, television, or poorly written online articles. It also stems from a lack of experience or pre-judgements about something a person may have only tried on one occasion.

We feel it is best to clarify what meditation is not, so you can better understand what it truly is to experience and appreciate its benefits.

1. Meditation is not about concentration; instead, it is about awareness.

For instance, during a Body Scan meditation you are asked to become aware of a particular body part, noticing any physical sensation in the area and then let go, meaning to relax that particular area and move onto the next.

During other meditations, people attempt to focus on one particular event, activity, emotion, or anything their energy and mind gives thought too. For the first few moments, this is effective because it causes a person to slow down their racing thoughts. However, if you continue to concentrate on something for too long, you will not gain any sense of awareness. Instead, realize the goal is to remain conscious of the present moment while no labeling or judging the thoughts in your mind.

2. Meditation is not a form of religious practice; rather it is a spiritual practice.

Without bringing up your feelings about religion, let us only look at the facts. In religious practices, there are rules and doctrines that dictate what to do, what you believe in, and how you live your life. With spirituality, you can create your journey in life, have your own perspective, and connect with your highest self. In essence, you are in control, and you don't need to consult with others on how to live.

3. Meditation is not about learning how to stop all of your thoughts completely.

Instead, it is about learning how to change our thought process altogether.

Have you ever gone through your day with endless self-talk? "Do this, don't do that, I'm the best, I'm the worst, you're going to be late, you're fat, I'm in horrible shape, I'm overweight... etc." All of these scattered thoughts are not our true selves. They are the result of a mind that is run by the ego.

Finding our true-self transpires when we can connect with that calmness within and we can "just be." Through meditation, we can significantly limit racing thoughts and transcend our minds.

4. Meditation is not weird; it's empowering.

Now this statement is more of an opinion than fact, but the belief for us remains true. We wouldn't publish this book if we didn't believe in the power of meditation. When people react negatively to a concept without having insight or knowledge, it is because they do not yet comprehend what they are criticizing. Our minds try to put a simple; easy to understand definition for every person and everything we encounter. We try to compartmentalize or put these concepts in a "box." However, most individuals, things, and concepts are more complicated than we can ever imagine.

Many do not realize what the real power of meditation can do and have yet to experience the calm and confident state of mind which comes from the practice. If a person labels meditation as "weird," it is also because they have not had the self-empowering feeling that comes from going deep within oneself. If they had, they would be telling everyone they know about how great they feel and how life changing it has been.

5.) You do not have to sit in the lotus position to meditate.

You may have seen somewhere on the internet or read in a section of a book that when it's time to meditate, you must sit in the lotus position (sitting in a cross-legged position with your palms on your knees facing up). Now, there is no denying this is a useful position because when your body sits up straight, it prevents you from falling asleep, and your energy can then flow up and down your body more effectively.

But make no mistake, the overall goal of meditation is to develop awareness and for some, that can come from lying down, standing up, or being in any position they desire. After our clients work out, we give them the option of identifying with their feelings to determine the position. If they feel tired and could fall asleep at any moment, the lotus position is a better option. If they have too much energy, lying down would be ideal.

When it comes down to it, it's all based on your needs at the time. Become aware of what's best for you and always trust your gut!

Chapter 7

HOW YOUR THOUGHTS AFFECT YOU

Throughout a typical day, we have a constant stream of thoughts racing through our minds. Research has shown that most of these thoughts are automatic and can have a profound impact on our lives. Have you ever been involved in a stressful situation and felt you had no control over the thoughts running through your mind?

In these situations, our fight or flight response kicks in giving us an increase in adrenaline. As a result, the ability to handle or be in control becomes nearly impossible.

What about something far less intense, such as when you look into a mirror and see your image staring back? What are the thoughts that go through your mind then? Are you saying to yourself, "Wow I look great" or is there just a persistent flow of one negative statement after another?

In both of these situations, we find our minds racing involuntarily and get so caught up in our thoughts that we feel out of control and insecure.

Additionally, worrying about the things we cannot control, being in environments with too much noise, remembering unpleasant memories from the past and overwhelming ourselves with too many commitments further contributes to our mental unrest.

For instance, when we over commit ourselves to a number of activities, we tend to fill up every second of our day with something to do. We are constantly on the go, bouncing from one activity to the next with no end in sight. Our minds are continuously thinking, and we never allow ourselves the opportunity to slow down and take a mental break.

With all of this exhaustion and mental depletion, we feel completely overwhelmed, stressed, and agitated. A simple solution, which we all struggle to employ, is the art of saying NO. This isn't always easy as with some commitments we have no other choice but to attend.

If we make an effort and take an honest and careful look at the multitude of things we are doing, we will start to realize which commitments are only causing us stress. Only you, yourself will know what is wasting your time, but more importantly, your precious and valuable energy. Be honest with yourself and start by cutting back on one commitment per week.

Now if we aren't overwhelmed with obligations and busy schedules, we are doing the complete opposite which is "worrying."

Worrying is a direct result of not taking action in regards to a problem and constantly thinking about the things that we cannot control.

Have you had this experience?

Whether worrying about the weather, the traffic, the economy or what others think or do, we must realize that some things are simply beyond our control. Believe it or not, not being able to control everything is a good thing. It takes away that overwhelming sense of responsibility and instead of worrying, it allows for a break to focus on the things that you can control while also letting go of what you can't control.

As previously mentioned, we will share with you a powerful exercise to assist you in letting go. Believe us when we tell you it is a powerful technique that when practiced, can transform your life.

But before we get there, let's talk about one of the reasons our minds race out of control which is: Being in environments with too much noise.

For instance, many of us turn on the television or put on music while performing an activity such as cleaning the house, driving, or spending time with our kids.

While music can be a source of motivation or give you the energy to work, you have to ask yourself "Is this background noise giving me mental unrest?" If you are going to listen to music, it is best to listen to something soft. From our experience, loud music tends to create a sense of unrest and overwhelms our minds, while soft music lets us fall into a gentle flow of conscious thought. Take our word for it; we wrote this book while listening to smooth jazz in Starbucks!

Even though learning how to alleviate stress is our goal, there are times where we simply can't control our environment. For example: being around screaming kids or being stuck in traffic with a person blasting their car radio next to us. Even in these overwhelming circumstances, we can use breathing techniques to slow down our mind and feel more in control. There are many variations of breathing you can perform to limit the racing thoughts. For us, especially in traffic, we like the 4-2-4 method.

The method involves breathing in for (4) seconds, holding that breath for (2) seconds and breathing out for (4) seconds. It's very simple and can take place anywhere. (If you are performing it in traffic, be sure to keep your eyes open.).

The next time you are in a stressful situation give it a try for (1) minute; you will notice a subtle yet powerful difference in the way you feel.

The last areas of self-defeating thoughts to discuss are unpleasant memories.

These memories usually arise unexpectedly, while other times they are brought on by none other than ourselves. For example, have you found yourself going through the Facebook page of someone you used to date or an old friend you've stopped talking too? For some reason, we find ourselves looking at their pictures and posts only to find all sorts of negative thoughts popping up in our head space.

Keep in mind this is something we can control. We have the power and ability to stop looking at others Facebook profiles, to remove them as a friend, or to get rid of any pictures we have of them. Our overwhelming stressors can be controlled, and it's important for us to do so when given the opportunity.

Negative Thought Patterns

After speaking and personally training hundreds of clients, we have learned from their experiences that if we don't have an overall positive view of ourselves, we will have an overwhelming amount of negative thoughts racing through our minds every day.

Our negativity can arise from a variety of sources. For some, it could be the negative thoughts about growing up in a household with parents who were negative or talked down to us. For others, it might be harmful or damaging life experiences. We don't deserve the bad things that happen to us, yet we feel a sense of responsibility for something beyond our control. It could have been a car accident, abuse from a loved one, or simply being in the wrong place at the wrong time.

How about our so called failures?

Depending on your outlook, we may try to achieve a goal such as putting yourself out there socially or attempting to try something new. If it doesn't go our way or exactly how you perceived it would, you become extremely frustrated and disappointed. When things don't go according to plan, you have two options. Either you take the event as a life lesson to learn from, or you internalize it as a failure. Unfortunately, most of us internalize these experiences as failures.

So how can we overcome all this negative thinking? How can we begin to change the way we think about ourselves and the world? How can we limit our racing and negative thoughts throughout the day?

The answer is something you may have never heard.

Are you ready for it....?

It's called shifting our FEELINGS!

Our feelings you ask? If you have heard of this concept, you're probably thinking something like, "Yeah, I already know that I heard it in the movie, The Secret." If that is you, hold on because I am going to share a technique to shift your feelings and truly let go so you can better enjoy the present moment and your life. For those new to this concept, let me explain how to shift your thoughts.

Earlier we mentioned that throughout the day, we have thousands of racing thoughts, most of which are negative and automatic. Since we can't control thousands of ideas, we need to shift our awareness to our feelings. When we focus on our feelings, we are in a better position to be in control of ourselves. For example, if we are thinking negatively while looking in the mirror, we could shift from a thinking perspective to that of an action perspective. We can choose to take action right then and there, such as a performing a couple of squats or pushups, and begin to FEEL our body at work. If we are stuck in traffic and getting agitated, we can listen to music to FEEL better.

You might say that is just suppressing, ignoring, or covering up the negative thoughts. However, as long as we can quickly acknowledge the thought such as, "I recognize I am negative right now but I want to change it," we can then shift our mindset without suppressing our emotions.

But what if you can't think of an action to take or have a feeling or thoughts that seem to consume you?

There is a solution; it's called the "The Letting Go" exercise.

The Letting Go Exercise

Have you ever had a particular thought you just couldn't get out of your head? Something you thought about over and over again to the point of distraction from work, school or your life's mission? It's happened to all of us and sometimes it feels like these thoughts consume our being. It might have been something we've done, something somebody has done or said to us, or something that started off as a minor problem. Regardless of what it was, the more we thought about this particular thing, the bigger the problem it became.

Typically, when these thoughts arise, we are never able to process them or let them go in a healthy manner. Instead, we either try to escape these thoughts by partaking in a vice, expressing them incorrectly or suppressing them. Suppressing isn't good for our mental or physical health, causing us to age prematurely or get sick. So how can we let go?

Thankfully, there is a simple 3 step technique you can do when you have a few moments to yourself. For safety purposes, be sure not to perform this technique while driving or operating heavy machinery.

The three step process can be broken down into:

1.) **Identify the problem**
2.) **Allow yourself to experience the problem (FEELINGS)**
3.) **Let it up and let it out**

Before applying this technique, we need to put ourselves in the best position for success. To do so, we must put ourselves in a state of awareness.

Find a comfortable place to sit, preferably a chair where you are sitting upright. You could sit down in the lotus position, but for this exercise, we prefer a chair with a straight back. Place your hands on your thighs with your palms facing up.

Keep in mind we need to feel fully present, and we need to ground ourselves. With your feet flat on the floor, picture roots sprouting out from your feet and going deep into the center of the earth. Picture them going deeper and deeper as your root yourself and become one with Mother Nature. Then, take your awareness to the bottom of your spine aka the Root Chakra. Be with this area and feel your body sinking into the chair.

Now, the first step we need to do is *Identify the Problem.*

Close your eyes and begin to become aware of your stomach. Begin to shift your thoughts to any feelings you may have in this area. Become aware of your gut feelings or what sensations are happening in this area around the Solar Plexus just around your belly button. If something is causing us stress we usually have some activity going on in this area; try to FEEL what is going on.

Second, allow yourself to experience the feelings and sensations without judgment. With awareness around your stomach, feel what is going on around there. It could be anxiety about a person or sadness about an event. There is no labeling, judgment, criticism, or any

thought from the mind. It is simply a feeling of awareness.

Begin to shift all your energy down to the base of your
spine. Allow your mind to empty as every feeling and
thought you have come down to this area. Even with
your breath, you want to bring it all down.

Once you have the feeling, begin the following:

Breathe in for 7 seconds, hold for 3 seconds, breathe out
for 7 seconds, hold for 3 seconds, and begin again. For
those familiar with Pyranic breathing, the technique is
6-3-6-3. Personally, we've found better success with our
clients with the extra second for breathing in and
breathing out. You will perform three cycles.

The Let Go Breath

With your awareness on your stomach:

Breathe in through your nose for 7 seconds
Hold for 3 seconds
Exhale through your mouth for 7 seconds
Pause for 3 seconds
Breathe normally for about 15 seconds

With your awareness on your stomach:

Breathe in through your nose for 7 seconds

Hold for 3 seconds
Exhale through your mouth for 7 seconds
Pause for 3 seconds
Breathe normally for about 15 seconds

With your awareness on your stomach:

Breathe in through your nose for 7 seconds
Hold for 3 seconds
Exhale through your mouth for 7 seconds
Pause for 3 seconds, then
Breathe normally for about 15 seconds

The next step is to let the feeling come up and out of you. This moment is where the magic happens and is an important step on the journey to healing ourselves

Once again you will perform the same breathing technique, however, this time, we want you to bring the feeling you have up during the inhale and then let it out fully during the exhale. Picture the feelings rising from the base of your spine and coming up and out of your mouth. These feelings have been identified from the previous round of breathing, and can now be let go.

Now, with your awareness on your stomach:

Breathe in through your nose for 7 seconds letting the feelings
rise up your body
Hold for 3 seconds
Exhale through your mouth for 7 seconds letting the feelings
out of your body

Pause for 3 seconds
Breathe normally for 15 seconds

Again, with your awareness on your stomach:

Breathe in through your nose for 7 seconds letting the feelings
rise up your body
Hold for 3 seconds
Exhale through your mouth for 7 seconds letting the feelings
out of your body
Pause for 3 seconds
Breathe normally for 15 seconds

One more time, with awareness on your stomach:

Breathe in through your nose for 7 seconds letting the feelings
rise up your body
Hold for 3 seconds
Exhale through your mouth for 7 seconds letting the feelings
out of your body
Pause for 3 seconds, then
Continue breathing normally

How do you feel now?

You should feel lighter, less tense, and more at ease
with yourself and the world. If there are still negative
feelings, you may need to repeat the cycle a few more
times. However, if you feel more at ease, congratula-
tions you are learning to let go! You have come to understand exactly how let go of all those feelings you
suppressed, wrongfully expressed or tried to escape.

Be sure to continue practicing this technique when you feel something is weighing you down or holding you back. You should perform this exercise every day so that your mind is always clear, calm and in control.

All things considered, the breathing technique you just learned is only one of the many that you can perform during meditation. Learning how to control your breath will not only change the way you feel about yourself, but it is the vehicle you need to be able to meditate properly.

Chapter 8

THE IMPORTANCE OF BREATHING

Breathing is a natural bodily function we all perform, without even thinking about it. Our bodies are intelligent as they control our breath through a system called the Autonomic Nervous System which almost completely acts unconsciously and also is responsible for our heartbeat and digestive process.[16]

Essentially, breathing is the most effective way to connect the mind and the body. When we consciously regulate our inhales and exhales, we can better control our mind and our emotions. In eastern philosophy, the belief is that breathing the correct way can help us live longer, increase our energy and help us to relax.[17]

If you ever observe someone sleeping soundly, you will notice that when they inhale their stomach expands deeply and when they exhale they lower their stomach back down. However, as busy individuals, we start to breathe in and out from our chest because of stress. This kind of breathing tends to be tense, erratic, shallow and all over the place. It causes the body not to become as fully oxygenated as if we were breathing from our lower abdominals.[18] Additionally, chest breathing does not allow us to relax and become fully present. This kind of breathing comes from an anxious state of mind, not that calm center we are trying to find.

When we begin to become aware of our breath we activate different parts of our brain, which can lie dormant. Typically, we operate from our reptilian brain or our brain stem, this area controls our automatic breathing. However, when we become consciously aware of our breathing, a different area known as the cerebral cortex is activated.

By controlling our breathing, the cerebral cortex can then balance and have a profound relaxing effect on our emotions. It does so by sending positive signals to the respiratory area in the mid-brain. From there, the impulses enter the hypothalamus which is an area corresponding to our emotions. The magnetic impulses sent to the hypothalamus then allow us to relax.

Types of Breathing

Within yoga and meditation, there are numerous techniques you can use to control your breathing and have a better sense of awareness. For simplicity purposes, we will only focus on four. One of which was created by us for our clients for them to let go.

As previously mentioned, the "Let Go Breath" involves: breathing in for 7 seconds, holding for 3, exhaling for 7 seconds and holding for three before repeating the same breathing pattern. We've found in our experience this is one of the most productive ways to enter a relaxed state of mind, let go of the emotions and mental chatter of the day as well as becoming more present. (Remember not to perform this technique while driving or operating heavy machinery.)

Simple Breath

Let us now explore other types of breathing techniques you can use in daily life. First, we will explore the Simple Breath, which is ideal for beginners as it teaches you how to breathe more deeply and develop a deeper sense of awareness. Also, it helps to reduce stress and anxiety as well as to better enter a flow state.

Choose a position that works best for you; it could be lying down on the ground, sitting upright in a chair or being in the lotus position. We always feel seated in a chair is your best option, but we encourage you to listen to your body and consider what is best for you. To begin, place one hand on your lower stomach and become aware of your breathing rate. Is your stomach rising fast and shallow or is it slow and relaxed? Just become aware of what is going on in your body, there is no need to change your breathing immediately.

After about 1-2 minutes, begin the Simple Breath meditation. With your eyes closed and your hand still on your lower stomach start to expand your stomach outwards as you inhale and let it come back as you exhale. Do not count any numbers just yet, instead, focus only on this technique for another 1-2 minutes.

When you find yourself more relaxed, begin the next step which is to incorporate numbers to count toward which will keep you focused and get you even more into that relaxed state. Begin using a 6-3-6-3 breathing technique.

Breathe in deeply for six seconds as your stomach expands, hold for three seconds, and then exhale as your stomach lowers back down, hold for three seconds. With this simple breath, you should find yourself calmer and much more relaxed than when you started.

The Cooling Breath

This form of breathing has profound effects on the body as it can decrease anxiety, improve concentration and reduce feelings of anger. The best time to use it is whenever you are feeling stressed, overwhelmed or agitated. During this breathing pattern, you will draw air across your tongue which almost feels like a cooling effect in your mouth.

Once again choose a position that works best for you, it could be lying down on the ground, sitting upright in a chair or being in the lotus position. As you know, we feel seated in a chair is your best option.

This form of breathing is more of an intermediate technique. First, with your eyes closed, clench your teeth and place your tongue gently against the back of your teeth. Begin to inhale through your clenched teeth all while making a hissing sound. Think back to when you may have touched a hot stove or a dish that hadn't cooled down; imitate the same hissing sound you would make during that situation. Once you have inhaled and held the breath, you will then exhale through your nostrils.

Yes, I know what you are thinking, " I thought it was always in through the nose and out through the mouth." A good point indeed, but for this technique, while counterintuitive, it will be our preferred method of breathing.

For this breathing technique, use a 4-2-4-2 method. Breath in through your clenched teeth for (4) seconds, hold for 2 seconds, exhale through your nostrils for 4 seconds and then hold for 2 seconds. You will begin to feel a cooling sensation in your mouth. Many of our clients have reported their breath had a cooling sensation and they felt very relaxed at the end of at this short breathing pattern.

The Long Exhale

The last breathing technique we want to share with you is called the "Long Exhale." This form of breathing is fantastic for those who struggle at night to fall asleep; it can improve problems with insomnia and like other forms of breathing it helps to control anxiety. We recommend using this breathing when you are lying in your bed, preparing to drift off to sleep.

To begin, place your hand on your stomach and start to count for how many seconds your body inhales naturally (stomach expanding) and then count how many seconds it exhales (stomach lowering).

Sometimes, when stressed, our inhaling breath is much longer than our exhaling breath. For this exercise, try to make both breaths equal, if you are breathing in for 3 seconds on the inhale naturally, begin to match that on the exhale. From there, focus on this new breathing pattern.

Once both your inhale and exhale are even, begin to extend the exhale by an extra 1-2 seconds. If you are comfortable inhaling for 3 seconds, start exhaling for 4 seconds. Then, when that feels comfortable, exhale for a total of 5 seconds. What you will find is that a slightly longer exhalation can produce a very noticeable and pleasant calming effect on your mind and body. By regularly practicing this form of breathing you will notice a great improvement in your overall quality of sleep.

Chapter 9

AWARENESS AND CONCENTRATION

Another reason so many people have a difficult time meditating is that they cannot find a sense of balance between concentrating and developing awareness. Concentration and awareness are two different functions of the mind, yet they are both still essential for meditation

Concentration is an energy that is singularly focused and directed toward one particular thing. As you begin to narrow your focus, its intensity, and power increase.

Have you ever seen a gymnast perform a routine?

They put such concentration into the routine they are about to perform. You can see it in their eyes, a laser-like focus.

They are concentrating on nothing but the routine they are about to perform. Whether it is the floor exercise,

Pommel Horse or balance beam, their concentration is at 10 out of 10.

How about studying for an exam or putting together a proposal at work, you know the more you concentrate on the work, the better the work will turn out.

During meditation, the act of concentrating is vital because it helps to slow down our racing minds. Instead of thinking about the craziness of the day or what we need to do, or what someone said to us, we can instead shift these thoughts into one particular person or object. By performing a body scan meditation, we re-direct our thoughts to a particular body part. This act alone is a form of meditation because a mind concentrating on just one thing enables us to relax. However, we need to be careful where we shift our focus. If we can keep our focus on a body part during a body scan meditation or our breath during a breathing exercise, we are using concentration for good.

However, being able to keep such an intense focus for a prolonged time during meditation requires that a person has the hours to practice to achieve such a goal.

Usually, our clients have reported maintaining great concentration for a minute or two, but then their thoughts shift toward something on a to-do list; something mean someone said to them, the argument they are currently in with their friends or spouse. Whatever it might be, there is a shift.

As you can see, concentration requires such a tremendous amount of will-power, which is difficult to sustain. In essence, it is a forced activity that will not give you a full perspective. Instead, it will keep things superficial.

While necessary for school, work or physical activities, it is also a starting point for meditation as it narrows your thoughts and slows a racing mind. But as you will also notice, we need more than concentration to reach an ideal state of mind. We need to bring in the other half, known as awareness.

Awareness differs from concentration because it observes what is passing through the mind and does not judge or label. Think of it as a river; it just flows with whatever is going through your mind.

While concentration cultivates itself through force, awareness develops from discovering your inner power. What we mean by this is there is not a significant action to take. Instead, it is a gentle effort in reminding ourselves that we need to let go and become aware. Earlier we shared with you a powerful exercise for letting go; we highly encourage you to go back and practice that exercise.

By gently reminding ourselves to become aware, we can be more present to the moment. As we persist in this simple effort, we begin to feel the depth to our meditation increase. We feel a sense of calmness take over, and we can just "be." Everything just feels right". It is a state of mind that can come and go, but with regular practice the depths of this feeling are limitless.

Chapter 10

BRINGING IT ALL TOGETHER: MIND & BODY

Developing the ideal balance of concentration and awareness is not impossible, and anyone can achieve this state. However, it does take consistent practice to hone this craft.

Typically, during the first few minutes of meditation, your mind will be racing with endless thoughts. As you have just learned, this is the ideal time to begin to concentrate on one particular thing. It could be a part of your body, a word, a feeling, whatever helps to keep you focused.

As you begin to develop a deeper sense of concentration, the question then becomes, "When do I shift to a feeling of awareness?"

This change is the key to getting the absolute most out of your meditation sessions. Too many people will spend their time only in the concentration state. They hyper-focus on something for so long that their concentration then manifests into either endless racing thoughts where they can't concentrate at all, or they turn into something we call "Statue syndrome" which is sitting like a statue without a thought or any sense of awareness. Think of it like you are "blanking out."

However, a person who immediately shifts into awareness without concentration becomes over stimulated. They begin to feel bombarded by everything. Their senses take on ADHD-like behavior, and the mind overwhelms itself with smells, noises, feelings and more. Picture a five-year-old child who just ate a big piece of cake while drinking a can of soda; that is what it is like to go into a full sense of awareness too soon.

So how do we find balance? What is the ideal time to shift our sense of concentration into a sense of knowledge for us to get the most out of our meditation?

The answer is quite simple; we need to find a state of calmness. We need to calm down our minds and be able to relax.

When you finally feel relaxed, that is when you can begin to become aware and experience the actual benefits of meditation. The best way we've found to achieve this calm feeling is to concentrate, specifically on your breathing.

As you can see, we have shared many different breathing techniques with you thus far, and we encourage you to go back and review those life changing breaths. Practice concentrating on your inhalations and exhalations. Pretty soon you will achieve that relaxed feeling. From there become aware and everything will finally feel "just right."

Once you feel confident that you have found this profound balance of concentration and awareness enabling you to enter deeper levels of meditation, we are ready to move on and discuss how you can use this ideal state of mind to change your life. Earlier you learned about the insider tips about how to lose weight and get in better shape. Next, we discussed how to meditate, its benefits and why it works so well after a workout. But now is the part you've all been waiting for.

You've put yourself through intense exercise; you've found a calm state through meditation. How do you now take it to the next level? How do you take it to a place where you FEEL absolutely fantastic about yourself? How do you bring your state of mind to the notion that every time you look in the mirror you FEEL good about yourself?

Get ready...

Because we are about to delve into the secrets of what makes our clients look and feel their absolute best.

PART III

AFFIRMATIONS

Chapter 11

THE LIFE CHANGING BENEFITS OF AFFIRMATIONS

After ten plus years of combined personal training experience, we have seen hundreds of clients hit their weight loss goals, tone their bodies, develop great core strength and improve their balance. For us, it is rewarding seeing people change their lives. However, while we saw the physical change, our clients never held on to the sustained sense of FEELING good.

For a short time, they would be happy when they hit a new low weight on the scale or finished a challenging workout. However, the next time we saw our clients there was always a nagging complaint about a flaw in their physical appearance or how they just felt.

Do you walk around every day of your life just feeling you're best?

Do you look in a mirror and always smile or do you

have some voice in your head telling you that you are not enough?

We all have this voice, and its presence and influence vary person to person. Our whole goal in writing this book is to minimize and eliminate this self-defeating thought process.

You've learned so far how to lose weight and tone muscles; then we covered how to calm your mind. Now let us explore what so many people struggle to bring into balance, "The Mind-Body Connection."

The term "Mind-Body" has become increasingly more popular over the last 10-20 years. The notion of being able to find a balance between the two has given rise to many yoga studios, countless self-development books, meditation retreats and more. We cannot minimize the power of the mind-body because it really can be so life-changing. The connection is something you need to experience, and each time you do, it becomes more profound.

Over the last ten years, I (Dan) have spent countless hours meditating, reading self-development books, performing Reiki on others and researching different meditation techniques. It wasn't until a few years ago that I realized the reason our clients were not feeling their best was that their mindsets were that of self-defeating thoughts, feelings, attitudes, and beliefs; I knew that this had to change. That is when I started to play around with meditations after fitness. The results were profound because I could see my clients beginning to feel better about themselves and their bodies. They weren't criticizing their bodies as much and were not complaining all the time that they were too heavy.

I noticed this pattern of confidence and happiness last for almost a week after the workout with meditation. However, I felt more could be done to help a person feel their best. It was at this point when I began to play around with affirmations.

The Power of Affirmations

The biggest and most profound changes for me and my clients took place when we began using affirmations. I started using them after a person had completed a workout and after they had found a sense of calmness and the ideal balance of concentration and awareness during meditation. It was at this point where the mind was most fertile and open to suggestion. It seemed when a person gets into this state; their egos are not in control, and it's almost like connecting with their true selves.

At some point in our lives, we're told we are not good enough from someone we know or love. It could be a certain phrase, a specific word or something subtle which didn't make us feel good. Combine that with the society in which we live is always promoting photoshopped images of "perfect people" that no one could ever become. Despite our best attempts to get the body we want and to feel good, we are always stifled and stopped by our minds past conditioning. It's frustrating, annoying and from our perspective, it just isn't right.

The only effective measure we have found to solve this problem was to speak positively about ourselves and others.

When we began implementing this technique, some of our clients started sobbing; some told us they hadn't heard anyone say something so positive to them in years. Then they talked about how good it felt to hear and feel the words settle into their minds causing them to feel happier and more alive.

As a result, we began using these affirmations with our clients on a full-time basis to make a dramatic change in the way they looked and thought about themselves. It caused a snowball effect of feeling better and better each time they looked into the mirror. It wasn't an ego driven sense of self; instead, it was a feeling of calmness and confidence in the mind-body; a belief in knowing that "I am enough."

Now, to begin to make changes for the better in the way we think and feel about ourselves, we need to begin to say affirmations to ourselves or hear the right kinds of affirmations. So many people believe they are saying positive things to themselves when in actuality they are just perpetuating the reoccurring negative thoughts and beliefs.

For instance, an individual who is trying to lose weight and use positive affirmations might say something like,

"I am no longer fat."

While this might sound like a step in the right direction, the real issue here is the word "fat." By using the word fat, they are giving it energy and allowing the word and everything associated with it to continue to exist. Instead, a better affirmation would be something like, "I have my dream body" or "My body is getting slimmer every day."

By changing the words of what we don't want to words of what we do want, we are laying the groundwork for dramatic change. Often as associated with the Law of Attraction, whatever we focus on continues to grow and remain present because we are giving it energy. By saying we are not fat we believe we will always be fat. By stating we are skinny, we are changing our thoughts, feelings, beliefs and attitudes toward a whole new way of life.

Overall, we have found there are five powerful types of affirmations we can say to ourselves or have others say out loud to us. Depending on the person, different affirmations will respond better based on your need.

Let's take a look at the types of affirmations below and see which resonate best with you.

1.) **Affirm what you want to have.**
    These kinds of spoken words address what you would like to look like, feel like or become. Think deeply about the dream body you want, what it would look like, what part you want to improve,

be sure to make the affirmation as descriptive as possible. "I am my dream weight, and I love my toned body, especially my.... "

2.) Affirm what you currently love about yourself.
For some, this might be difficult, especially if we are in a place where we feel awful about ourselves. Try to dig deep and think of some quality you like about yourself. It could be something physical such as your eyes, hair, hands or more importantly it could be a personality trait. It might be you are a good listener, a hard worker or even that you are a person who is dedicated to better their lives. You did purchase this book after all! Say something like..."I love how dedicated I am to losing weight, and it shows how mentally tough I am."

3.) Affirm you are in control.
Many of us point the blame toward others when in reality we are the ones to blame. We blame society, our family, fast food restaurants, anything as to why we aren't looking and feeling our best. However, when we take ownership of our problems, we can then empower ourselves. We can enhance our ability to take control of our lives by saying something like, "I choose/decide to take responsibility for my health." "I will workout (x) numbers of days per week," "and I will meditate after each workout."

4.) Affirm that you know.

Do you believe you can do something or do you KNOW you can do something? If we say we believe something will happen, we have some faith it might come to fruition. However, by only "believing," in something, we are giving our power away. Instead, we want to "know" it's going to happen. By knowing we put the control back in our hands because we can dictate what choices we make in our lives. A great affirmation here would be, "I know I will weigh (x) by (this month), or I know I'm going to make my goal (x).

5.) Affirm that you are grateful.

It might sound like a cliché, or something you hear in all self-development books, but being grateful does shift your perspective on how you feel about yourself and others.

If we don't express gratitude, our egos take over, and we become selfish. When we aren't thankful for our bodies, for instance, we tend to resent or feel unhappy about our self-image, even more.

Using affirmations are important because it can make us love our bodies even when we aren't at our ideal weight. By loving our bodies now, we will love our image even more, especially when we hit our goals.

Too many times people say I will be happy when

I'm this weight or fit into this outfit. If you aren't grateful now, you will always be chasing happiness. It's an endless cycle. Try being grateful, say, "I am so happy and thankful for my body and its ability to get through these workouts."

Chapter 12

WHAT YOU SHOULD SAY TO YOURSELF

As you have just seen, there are five different ways of using affirmations. When first starting out we suggest using, "Focusing on what you want to have."

This statement will make a life-changing difference in the way you think and feel about yourself. If you are a beginner, don't overwhelm yourself, keep it simple and stick with just one affirmation.

During our meditations with clients, we tend to use all five types of affirmations to varying degrees. Below are more examples you can use during your affirmations:

1.) **Affirm what you want to have.**
"I am slim and toned."
"I am muscular and thin."
"I weigh (x), it's my ideal weight."
"I can fit into those pair of pants."

"I am healthy and have lowered my cholesterol."

2.) Affirm what you currently love about yourself.
"I love how dedicated I am to losing weight."
"I love how good I feel after working out."
"I love how I am finally taking time for myself."
"I love how I am eating much healthier now."
"I love my body."

3.) Affirm you are in control.
"I decide when I workout."
"I choose to be happy."
"I choose to eat healthy foods."
"I choose to feel good about myself."
"I decide how to feel around others."

4.) Affirm that you know.
"I know I will weigh (lbs/kg's) by (date)"
"I know that my body is getting stronger every day."
"I know my body is getting leaner every day."
"I know I can choose to feel happy at any time."
"I know meditation helps me feel in control and calm."

5.) Affirm that you are grateful.
"I am so happy and grateful for my body."
"I am so happy and grateful for delicious, healthy food."
"I am so happy and grateful for my workout time."
"I am so happy and grateful for finding time to meditate."
"I am so happy and grateful now that I look and feel my absolute best."

Ideally, we love to combine all the aspects into one paragraph.

After months of meditation and practice we have our clients say:

"I am on pace for reaching my ideal body weight of (x). I love how focused I am on becoming skinny; it shows how much will power I possess. I choose to take responsibility for my health by working out (x) days per week. I know I will weigh (x) by the end of (x). Most importantly, I am so happy and grateful now that I have made the choice to look and feel my absolute best."

The best time to use these affirmations is after your workout and during your meditation when you have reached a state of calmness. The question then becomes how do I get these words into my head to reprogram my subconscious? Should I think them in my head or should I listen to them out loud? You could say them to yourself out loud or to yourself in your head.

However, an even more powerful way to experience and let these words resonate is to listen to them via a voice recording.

Chapter 13

THE POWER OF AUDIO AFFIRMATIONS

When allowing a deep state of meditation to take place, we find ourselves in a state of calmness and a feeling of bliss overtakes us because our mind can finally relax. The mind is not racing or thinking about the craziness of the day. It isn't thinking of the next thing to do; it is simply happy and at peace.

So how then do we get powerful, life-changing affirmations into our heads so we can re-program our subconscious to look and feel our absolute best?

One such option is to have somebody speak affirmations to us out loud. It could be a personal trainer, a close family member or a friend. We've found the powers of spoken words on audio recordings are even more life changing then saying affirmations in our heads when we first start this process.

As you will hear with the guided meditations on our YouTube Channel "The Mind Body Melt," we have two stages of affirmations. The first have to do with us saying the words, "You are..."

The "You Are" meditations are the first step and are ideal for beginners. These meditations with affirmations are for people new to this practice because receiving a compliment or approval from another person is much easier and impactful then by giving ourselves the affirmations. We are so conditioned not to think highly of ourselves, that the positive words of another make the greatest impact at first.

Over time we start to realize while others words can be quite influential, we soon discover our words are all that matters. The things others say to us can have an impact on how we feel, yet nothing is stronger than our own words.

Are you ready to take it to the next level?

To do so, you must speak the words yourself into a voice recorder app.

"You expect me to do what? But I hate my voice!"

There is no doubt listening to a guided meditation can transform your life. Having someone else guiding you into a state of relaxation and listening to affirmations about you can make an enormous impact in the way you look and feel about yourself.

So often in life, we are told we are not enough in some

shape or form. It could be someone blatantly putting us down or simply ignoring us. As humans, we are social creatures and crave the approval of others at the deepest layer of our core. When others think positively of us, and we hear their words of validation, it makes us feel great.

But what does it take to get even better results?

As you will see on our channel, there are more intermediate and advanced levels of meditations with affirmations. Once we guide you into a state of deep relaxation, you will notice the affirmations begin to shift from "You are" into "I am." We have you repeat the words "I am" followed by the rest of affirmation.

What's the difference?

Having someone tell us, "You are this..." or "you are that" has a profound impact on our lives. It can mold and shape us into a person we want to be, or we could become someone we despise. When we say the words, "I am" we are taking ownership of ourselves and our lives. By saying "I am," we are telling our brains, the only person's opinion that matters are mine. No one can tell me who I am, what I can do, or how to act. I control my life and decide what is best for me.

Saying the words, "I am" does one of two things.

First, it enables your Reticular Activation System or your RAS to engage. This part of your brain will focus more on whatever you tell it.[19] For instance, if I say don't focus on a yellow car, what does your mind start to think about?

How about for just one day you start to pay attention to all of the red Ford Mustangs on the road. All of a sudden you see red Mustangs everywhere. Seeing the SUV demonstrates the power of the RAS and when we use the words "I am" your mind will search high and low to find more evidence to support this statement. So if you say I am fat, your mind will find a way to reinforce this thought. It could be through eating bad foods, making excuses not to exercise or feeling badly about yourself. However, if you say "I am healthy," your RAS will look for ways of reinforcing that you are healthy. You will want to go to the gym, eat better foods and you will start to feel good about yourself.

Similar to your RAS, the Law of Attraction (LOA) is also quite impactful to your life. While the "RAS" is from western science, the LOA comes from theories of quantum physics. Numerous books written over the years discuss the power of the law of attraction. We, ourselves believe in the LOA and how what you focus on expands. Whatever the mind believes and conceives it can achieve. The movie, "The Secret" states, if you ask and believe you shall receive. Whether you think one or both of these concepts are valid, there is no denying the power of "I Am." Whatever you tell yourself that "you are," will set you on a course of what you claim to be.

As you can see the word, "I Am" is powerful. If you've paid attention, you've noticed that the affirmations on our YouTube Channel and from this book involve us telling you that "You are" or "I am" as part of the affirmation. Understand that listening to these words from another is essential for any beginner before moving onto more intermediate and advanced levels of meditations with affirmations.

Given this information, one has to think, could I take affirmations to an even more profound level of understanding?

Yes, you can!

Let us go further down the rabbit hole.

The reason we need to use guided meditations with affirmations from another's voice at first is that for one reason or another we don't believe our words. Instead, we look to others to tell us how to think and feel.

However, if another person has the same thought we almost always believe it to be true. The reason this happens is that we haven't developed into a self-assured individual. We haven't found some level of self-actualization. As the saying goes, "Know thyself." We may think we know, but do we?

Before this gets too confusing, let's take a step back.

Simply put, if you can create your voice recorded affirmations, you will have found the ideal way to make a life changing impact on the way you look and feel about yourself.

If you don't truly feel happy about your self-image and your mindset, it can be difficult to start feeling better about yourself on your own. Your brain will dismiss the affirmations as false, stupid, and a waste of time. It takes effort, time and a willingness to go within. But make no mistake about it, when you get to that next level, you will start to believe in your own words. Better yet, by knowing your words to be the truth, you will have made a jump to a positive place few people will ever know.

After years of practicing these meditations with affirmations, I (Dan) have found myself to be happier and happier every single day. I have never felt so good about myself, and I mean that with all honesty. The opinion of others doesn't bother me one bit, whether it be criticism or a compliment, it just is what it is. This new mindset doesn't mean I ignore everyone who's critical, or that I am not grateful for a compliment, rather it means only I can control how I think and feel. Only I can tell myself what I am, who I am and what I want out of life. I finally got to this place when I was able to progress to the level of voice recording my own affirmations and playing them when I obtained a calm state of mind during meditation.

When creating my voice recordings, I had to consider the words I was speaking into my I Phone. As we've discussed, whatever we focus on expands and our brains will search for evidence of it. As a result, I knew I had to stay away from sayings like, "I am not fat, "I am no longer weak, "I am happy not to be out of shape, "I am no longer depressed, or "I no longer feel bad about myself." However, if I had used the words: fat, weak, out of shape or depressed with my affirmations, I would have given those words energy and they would have manifested in some way. For example, I would still be depressed, out of shape or fat.

Instead, the affirmation needed to be straightforward and positive. I began using words such as "I am in shape, "I am happy and in love with my body, "I love how muscular and thin I am" "I feel amazing, life is great." These were the affirmations I used on my journey. I encourage you to do the same. Sit down and write what you want to be or what you have become. Whether or not you are at your ideal body weight, toned, happy, whatever physical or emotion it might be, believe and know who you are at this moment. You will activate your RAS or the LOA to make this thought a reality. Remember, thoughts become things!

Playing your Audio Affirmations

From everything we've discussed thus far, we know the best time to play our audio recording of affirmations is during our meditations when we feel a state of calmness. It is when we will make the most impactful change to our lives. We cannot stress enough the profound changes it has made in our lives and the clients we've trained throughout the years.

You might be thinking, well that sounds great, but what

if I can't get to this level of calmness during meditation?

Have no fear because these affirmations can still make an impact. If you have difficulty meditating, play them after you have performed a physical activity. By exercising and then listening to affirmations, even without that sense of calmness, the words will still enter into your sub-conscious.

But what about on days when I don't work out?

If you are unable to exercise due to the absurd trivialities of life, listen to your audio recording first thing in the morning. During this time, your brain is most at ease, listening to these words can set a tone for the day in how you think and feel.

What if I sleep late or can't exercise that day?

If you're having one those days, you can still receive some benefit from the affirmations. Play them while parked in your car, in between meetings or even listen to them in the bathroom. It doesn't matter where it occurs; just find the time to hear your powerful words.

Ideally, a recorded affirmation session will last for around 5 to 10 minutes. We recommend you starting with a 5-minute session and then build up to 10 minutes as you gain patience and start to feel a change overtake you. Some of our clients will go up to 15 or 20 minutes. This increase isn't necessary unless you have the time to do so. Five to ten minutes has been shown to be the ideal and most efficient time to get what you need.

Listed on the next page are some useful tips you can use when creating your affirmations:

1. Start by making a list of everything you want to have in the next few months. It can be your ideal weight, toned, muscle, peace of mind, calmness. Whatever it is, make a list of at least five different things you want to be.

2. Next, make a list of 3 things you currently love about yourself. Be honest and ask friends or family what they love about you.

3. Third, make a list of what you have some control over in your life and the decisions you can make. For instance, "I decide to be happy" or I am in control of my nutrition, or "I work out (x) days per week.

4. Fourth, create a list affirming what you know to be true. "I know I am becoming skinnier each week" "I know I am becoming healthier," etc.....

5. Fifth, create a gratitude list. For example, "I am grateful for my healthy body, I am so happy and grateful for becoming leaner."

6. Find a voice recorder or use a recording device on your smartphone. If you have the "Iphone," you can ask Siri to "Open Voice Recorder".

7. Record your affirmations. Find a quiet place in your house or your car by yourself. Say them slowly but with a powerful voice. When you say these words, you should feel the magnitude behind them. I know you're probably still thinking, "I hate listening to my voice." Don't worry; you will see in a little bit the power behind recording your voice.

8. Make each list of affirmations go for 1 minute. For instance, the list of what you want to be, speak those statements slowly yet powerfully until 1 minute has passed, then move on to the next list.

9. Congratulate yourself on a job well done. You have taken an important step in changing your life.

10. Listen to your audio recording for 5 minutes daily. At first, you might cringe hearing your own voice, but after a while you will begin to love your voice. You will feel empowered and look forward to hearing yourself speak highly of yourself. For one reason or another, we don't like to hear our voice. But by beginning to listen to yourself, you will start to assume a new and enlightened view of who you are.

Chapter 14

MIROR, MIROR ON THE WALL

One of the driving forces behind writing this book was that we wanted our clients, as well are ourselves to look and feel our absolute best. No better example of our critical judgment of ourselves comes when we look in the mirror. For one reason or another, every time we see our reflection we immediately begin to find something that isn't perfect. It might be societal conditioning from Hollywood or our parent's subconscious influence Whatever it is we are overly critical trying to compare ourselves to some ideal image of perfection which does not exist.

After performing hundreds of hours of research on the internet, we found people look at themselves in a mirror between 8-10 times per day[20]; and that is just in a mirror. Other studies which included any reflection such as a window, water or smartphone found it can be up to 60 to 70 times per day.[21] By performing our own naturalistic research in the field of life, we believe it to be much higher. During our training sessions with clients, we caught them looking at themselves at least 15 times not including when they were looking to check out their form.

Since we glance at ourselves so often, doesn't it make sense that our thoughts and feelings during this time should be positive and uplifting?

Of course, they should!

But let us delve even deeper into this topic…

Do you remember yourself as a child staring at yourself in a mirror for more than a minute or two?

Most of us have, and it has been quite an experience. After gazing at ourselves for a few minutes, interesting thoughts begin to pop up in our heads. As the famous author Paulo Coelho says, "The eyes are the mirror of the soul and reflect everything that is hidden; and like a mirror, they also reflect the person looking into them." Now we don't want to lose you if you think we are getting a little woo-woo here so, try to stay with us.

Whether or not you believe we have souls isn't a discussion we are trying to start. Instead, we are simply pointing out that when we look into a mirror, especially into our eyes, we begin to see depth. There seems to be more than meets the eye. By looking at ourselves, we can start to find answers. It's almost like we are finally facing our true-selves and giving ourselves an honest look. From there, we can find answers to our most nagging problems.

Remember the Michael Jackson song, "Man in the Mirror?" The song is about him looking into a mirror and realizing he needs to make a change. He wants to make a change for the better, and when he comes to this mirror, he is honest with himself. He understands to make this happen; he needs to start with himself.

Personally, we enjoy having our clients look in the mirror and tell us what they see reflected back. Once the initial negative judgments have been verbalized, we have them softly gaze at themselves. It's amazing to see how after about 3-5 minutes of self-defeating talk, we see a shift in perspective. They begin to talk about deeper issues than just how they look. They speak to things they have been putting off, goals to work toward and things they want to accomplish.

Try this for yourself, go to your nearest mirror take a look at yourself. For this exercise, you can verbalize whatever comes to mind for the first 1-3 minutes. It's typically frowned upon when people say negative things to themselves, but for this exercise don't worry about it. In a bit, we will show you a process of steps to speak positively to yourself. But for now, rid yourself of those self- defeating impulses and thoughts.

After three minutes of looking into the mirror, begin to gaze softly at your reflection. Look into your eyes and see the depth of color in your eyeballs; notice your pupils. Are they getting bigger or smaller? Begin to let any remaining thoughts go and just become aware. Become aware of how you feel. The rest is your personal experience, try not to freak out, but look at yourself for as long as you feel comfortable. You are now looking at your true-self; you will find answers to your most nagging problems. Write down what you've found and begin to make the necessary changes.

Stop reading right where you are right now and give this a try. Only continue reading on once you've looked at your reflection.

Now be honest, how did you feel during the first few minutes? Did you feel good or bad about yourself when speaking? What was on your mind?

While this is a powerful exercise, we want to share with you a different approach to getting more in touch with your true self.

So far you have learned the power of affirmations and how they can influence your sub-conscious and transform your life. Before we start combining affirmations and a mirror, let's start with something simple. The next time you look in a mirror, we want you to do just one thing.

Are you ready for it?

We want you to SMILE.

"Oh wow, ground breaking stuff" you might be thinking with a sarcastic voice!

But think about this...

Too often we look in the mirror, especially in the morning with a look of disgust. It could be subtle or blatantly obvious, but we heard it with our clients and we used to see it with ourselves. To begin changing for the better, we want you to start smiling but not just any smile.

The smile you are going to start using is what we call a Mona Lisa smile.

Have you ever looked at the famous painting by Leonardo da Vinci? Take a look and notice how she is smiling. She isn't giving a big cheesy smile, and she isn't giving a fake smile we so often do when we see someone we do not like, yet still feel the need to be friendly. Instead, the Mona Lisa smile is subtle yet powerful. It is an expression which projects confidence from the inside out. It says, I am confident, I know who I am and what I want out of life. At least that's our interpretation, but be-sure to give her smile another look and you will see exactly what we mean.

Begin by flashing a Mona Lisa smile to yourself every time you look in the mirror. For as long as your eyes are looking in the mirror, you are smiling like her. You will begin to notice your thoughts, feelings, attitudes and beliefs about yourself begin to shift when performing this simple task.

Now, if you want to make the most out of the mirror, use the smile, while listening to your audio affirmations.

As you have learned the most powerful way to use your affirmations is after a workout and during meditation when you reach a state of calmness. However, this type of sub-conscious re-programming is something else you could do to reinforce your new image. It might seem a little odd, and you might not be ready for it for quite some time. But know that it is there for you as a way to change how you look and feel about yourself. When you smile like this, you will not only feel amazing about yourself, but your true-self will shine through.

Chapter 15

UNLOCKING YOUR TRUE POTENTIAL

We want to give you the highest praise for deciding enough is enough. For realizing there is something you can do to make a change in your life and that you deserve to be happy.

Throughout your life, you've always been searching for something outside of you to make you feel good about yourself. Deep down a part of you always knew that the only person's opinion that matters most is your own. You've seen others go through life with ease and with a high level of confidence. You've had moments and times when you felt the same way.

 You know there is a way to make this feeling more of a permanent reality than a fleeting moment. You know you deserve to live the life you want to live. You know there is more to life than your current mental, emotional, physical and spiritual state.

The only thing you've been missing is the right formula. That is until now. With this system, you now know the right action steps to take; three things you knew existed but never knew to combine.

With The Mind Body Melt, you now have your guided path to take you to where you want to go.

It looks like this:

- **Exercise** Using High Intensity Interval Training
- **Meditate** After your workout
- **Affirm** the person you want to be.

This simple, yet highly effective system can show you how to live a healthier and more enjoyable life. It can inspire you to take action and become the best version of yourself. Remember, it all starts with you waking up and realizing there is so much more you can be, have and do.

It took me, (Dan) almost 15 years of meditating, reading numerous self-development books, studying four years of undergraduate classes in Psychology, two years of graduate study in Rehabilitation Counseling, four years of Reiki, 5+years of personal training and constant trial and error with my clients and with myself.

It took Rob and his 6+ years of hands on personal training as well as 15+ years of motivational selling in the corporate world for this formula to come to fruition. We are so happy to be able to share our work with you. Millions of people will exercise, meditate and use affirmations. However, none of them know how to effectively combine all three of them into a proven system to look and feel your best.

That is until now; now it's your turn.

My friend,

You are so close to looking and feeling your absolute best, not only when looking in the mirror, but throughout your everyday.

You're willing to make this feeling more of a permanent feeling than a fleeting moment.

You just need to realize you deserve this.

Your door of opportunity has just opened, walk through it!

Refuse to let your past feelings of self-doubt, self-consciousness, and self-defeating behaviors hold you back. They were experiences from the past and now is the present time. Learn from the past and transform yourself, elevate yourself to the next level.

Throughout our lives we worry about how much we weigh, how stressed we are and how we feel about ourselves, and we go through stretches where we are just stuck. We feel like a ship without a compass.

But, eventually something helps steer the ship; something gets us back on track. This time, it's *The Mind Body Melt*, a proven success system that can be a life-long motivator, inspirer, and friend.

In one year from now where do you want to be?

Do you want to be a happy, self-confident person who radiates positivity everywhere you go because deep down inside you know you are enough; and that you, yes you are the creator of your character and your world?

If you want to embody and become this person, it is up to YOU! There is always somebody out there in a worse situation than you and who's had even worse experiences happen whose overcome their demons and has succeeded. We are living proof it's possible. We used to look in the mirror and feel not so great about ourselves. Now, we look and feel fantastic.

Start your journey at once; do not let anyone hold you back. Don't let an unsupportive friend; doubtful spouse or even you stop you from becoming the person you want to be.

Your journey starts with beginning your HIIT training. Be sure to check out our YouTube Channel for free workouts, or you can purchase our high-quality full-length 6-week workout program on our website: www.TheMind-BodyMelt.com

During these workouts, we spend time with you taking you through each step of the process. From there you will learn the how to meditate; you'll let the stress of the day melt away, and your mind will become relaxed and calm. When your mind is calm, you can then listen to or speak your affirmations. The rest will take care of itself.

This is your best opportunity to look and feel your absolute best. Begin using the three step formula of fitness, meditation and affirmations to become the best and happiest version of you. We know you can do it!

You've just discovered a unique, but proven system for finally re-discovering the self-confidence you know you have. It's no accident you are here. Your efforts and thoughts have guided you toward us, and we are so happy to give you the tools you need to be successful.

The time is now. We have given you everything you need to succeed. We are so excited for you and the person you will become. Take the step and begin at once. We KNOW you can do it.

PART IV: THE ACTION PLAN

Bonus # 1

THE 30 DAY MIND-BODY MELT CHALLENGE

To make the changes to become the person we want to be, we must take action. To help you get to there, we've created a simple 30-day action plan to help you start your journey. The program is broken down into days 1-10, 11-20 and 21-30.

In the next chapter, you will learn the action steps to develop the confidence to inspire real change without feeling overwhelmed. As you continue along your journey, you will find yourself enjoying exercise as well as meditation and affirmations. Eventually, you will think to yourself, "Why haven't I done this before?"

We have seen clients successfully change their habits in as little as 21 days. However, we've seen even better and longer sustained changes from those who took the full 30-day challenge. These individuals were able to move into what we call the empowered stage of change.

Day 21 is where they get a taste of empowerment, by day 30 they embody empowerment.

So what does this mean?

From years of experience coaching our clients, applying theories of psychology and reading countless books on habits, we've created a 30- day beginners guide that speaks to what it takes to make a positive change in a person's life.

Here is what it looks like:

Days 1-10. Exhausted

Days 11-20 Encouraged

Days 21-30 Empowered

EXHAUSTED

During the first 1-10 days of taking on any new habit, we can find ourselves beyond exhausted. Yes, the first day or two we might be highly motivated and excited about the changes soon to be experienced; but since motivation is fleeting, we cannot sustain our excitement. After a few days, we find ourselves exhausted, making excuses and falling back on our bad habits. We might eat something unhealthy, find an excuse not to work out, say we don't have the time or think we are unworthy of changing ourselves.

The first 1-10 days is about testing our will-power and finding the strength to push through. Over the years our habits have been conditioned, which make our limiting beliefs seem too overwhelming to continue on this 30-day challenge.

Don't give up!

Recognize what's going on, focus and begin to visualize the person you want to become. If you continue to concentrate on your goals, you will make it through these challenging first ten days. Once you've made it through, you will begin to feel a sense of **encouragement.**

ENCOURAGMENT

After ten days, you will start to feel different. You might not have the body of your dreams right now, but you will feel much better about the direction where you are heading. In a matter of just a few days, you will have developed an increased sense of confidence and others will start to notice that you seem a little bit happier.

The feeling can be exhilarating!

However, this is where many people end up self-sabotaging themselves. With this new feeling, your ego will begin to talk to you. You still start to hear voices saying, "I don't need this anymore I feel better or "I've been good the last 10+ days, I'll take a day off." Become aware of this voice and immediately take your action steps that day if you haven't done so already.

During days 11-20 you have made progress, but you haven't fully developed your new habit. You are well on your way and are far ahead of those struggles you faced for the first ten days.

Keep moving forward; you can't give up, and you can't give in. You've come so far; you need to hold on because soon you will experience an even more satisfying feeling known as **Empowerment**.

EMPOWERMENT

Ah yes, a feeling we all wish to have.

As you finish your 21st day in a row of *The Mind Body Melt* Challenge, you will transition from "doing" the action steps to becoming the "change" you wish to be. Because you took action for three weeks in a row, you have now become a person who exercises, meditates and speaks highly of themselves through affirmations.

Day 21 is a powerful day, but don't stop here. Continue for the full 30 days to fully develop the new habit and the new you. After 30 days you will feel like an empowered and unstoppable force. Your confidence and self-esteem will have never felt better.

When you realize you can change your mind and your body in such a short period, you will begin to think, "What else can I change?" It could be your finances or your relationships; it's totally up to you. We believe the mind and body are of the biggest challenges anyone can undertake. Once you get these two areas of your life under control, everything else is relatively seamless.

Remember, we started off slowly to build confidence. Don't try to change the steps we have created for you. For some, it might seem that this is way too easy, others might feel overwhelmed. The primary goal during these first 30 days is to build the new habit. After 30 days, you can add on even more time for exercise, increase the length of your meditation, increase the number of affirmations and eat more vegetables.

Now, without further ado, let's take a look at just what it will take to become the new you:

Days 1-10 (Perform each of the following once a day for ten days.)

Eat **1** Green Vegetable

5 Minutes of High-Intensity Interval Exercise (Day 1,3,5,7,9)

5 Minutes of Jogging, Walking Running (Day 2,4,6,8,10)

1 minute of Breathing and Meditation each day.

1 minute of saying one positive affirmation to yourself each day.

Days 11-20 (Perform each of the following once a day for ten days.)

Eat **2** Green Vegetables

10 Minutes of High Intensity Interval Exercise (Day 11,13,15,17,19)

10 Minutes of Jogging, Walking Running (Day 12,14,16,18,20)

2 minutes of Breathing and Meditation each day.

2 minutes of saying two positive affirmations to yourself each day.

Days 11-20 (Perform each of the following once a day for ten days.)

Eat **3** Green Vegetables

15 Minutes of High Intensity Interval Exercise
(Day 21,23,25,27,29)

15 Minutes of Jogging, Walking Running (Day 22,24,26,28,30)

3 minutes of Breathing and Meditation each day.

3 minutes of saying three positive affirmations to yourself each day.

Right now you might have numerous questions racing through your mind. What kinds of vegetables should I eat? What kind of workout should I perform for High-Intensity Interval Training? Is there a particular breathing technique I should use? What should the affirmations be?

Take a breath and let's take a look.

Bonus # 2

SPECIFICS OF THE 30-DAY CHALLENGE

Don't worry about the size of the vegetables, or any other specifics. The goal is to eat one green vegetable for the first ten days. The benefits of eating vegetables are immense, in fact, whole books have been written just on that topic.

For our sake let's keep it simple, eat one vegetable for the first ten days. Believe us when we tell you, you will begin to notice its benefits.

Some of us are already doing this, but for many, there can be days or weeks that go by before the benefits manifest themselves. It's as if your body is going through a detoxification process. We feel its best if you choose which meal you eat your vegetables, but to start, we recommend having them with dinner.

In no particular order, here are some of our recommendations: *kale, spinach, romaine lettuce, collard greens, Swiss chard, cucumbers, and broccoli.* Be sure to perform a google search for more ideas.

Types of Workouts

As you begin exercising, you will notice some days you are performing HIIT training while other days you are exercising by engaging in some cardio. We love HIIT training, but if you are doing it every day for 30 days, you are going to burn yourself out or possibly injure yourself, especially if you are new. Use the even numbered days for some form of cardio which can include: walking, jogging, running or even jumping jacks.

These don't have to be performed at a vigorous pace. The goal is to get your body moving. Ideally, you will be outside, performing your cardio in a safe environment. Walking around a mall or engaging in jumping jacks at home is always an alternative if need be.

There are many sources of information on YouTube and through Google searches where you can find HIIT workouts from fitness professionals. Be sure to find programs which focus on strength training and cardio.

We highly recommend you check out our YouTube Channel, The Mind Body Melt, where we post free Workouts of the Week. These workouts deliver heart pumping, calorie burning and muscle toning results in less than 30 minutes a day. We update the channel weekly, so there are always new and exciting exercises for you to choose. Best of all, you decide how many rounds to perform. We give you the option to do as little as one or as many as five to make the most out of your time.

Remember, don't overdo it. We recommend a total of 2-4 HIIT workouts per week. The off days are yours to do whatever you like such as walking, jogging, sprinting, jumping jacks, etc.

If you want to maximize your time and get the best results even faster, be sure to check out our website, www.TheMind-BodyMelt.com. There you will find a 6-week holistic fitness program where you get to work out, meditate and listen to affirmations with us. We are there every step of the way to coach, guide and support you in making the change to looking and feeling your best.

Wherever you find your HIIT workout, be sure to print it out, screen shot it or write it down and store it in a place where you know you won't lose it. Follow the exercises in order as recommended and push yourself to the point where you can feel your heart rate elevate and feel sweat dripping from your brow. We recommend using HIIT workouts because they give you a full body workout.

Types of Breathing and Meditation

Throughout this book, you have learned a few breathing exercises you can perform during your meditations which include: The Simple Breath, The Cooling Breath, and the Long Breath. Your initial thought might be to perform the simple breath for the first ten days, then the cooling breath for days 11-20 and finish with the long breath for the last ten.

While this might seem logical, we found it best for each person to assess their development. For instance, it took us months to feel comfortable using the simple breath before advancing to the cooling breath. Your ego will tell you that you need to learn everything at once and that you "got this." Be sure to trust your intuition and assess whether you are ready to progress.

We highly recommend you stick to the simple breath for the first 30 days. You will notice your mastery of this breath will increase with each day of practice. Feelings of anxiety will reduce, and you will be able to relax a little quicker each time. You'll soon gain confidence with each session and will be able to let go of whatever is on your mind.

Don't be hard on yourself if you feel you aren't ready to advance to the cooling breath right away. It isn't a race; it's a journey of self-development. Wherever you are is where you are meant to be. Be happy with your progress and smile knowing that you are becoming a better person each day.

Types of Affirmations

Properly using affirmations is one area where many of our clients get stuck. Many begin to start overthinking and ask, "Do I use my voice? Do I just say it to myself in my head? Do I have someone else say these affirmations?

There is no one size fits all answer. Just like the breathing exercises, it will depend on your personal preference. However, we can share with you what works most efficiently with our clients.

First, we highly recommend you start by using an audio tape recording. The reason for this is that, while we try to say nice things to ourselves after meditating in our heads, we instead have self-defeating thoughts. Our minds start off with good intentions, but then we start to doubt what we are saying, we think of past experiences that might not validate this new positive thought, or our minds begin to wander.

Instead, have somebody you know speak the affirmation for you. Make sure it is someone who is supporting you on your journey and that you know has your best intentions in mind. For instance, we spoke the affirmations for our clients into their smartphones. If you don't have a personal trainer, find that one person in your life that is supportive. It could be a family member, a friend, a religious leader, a coworker, ideally anyone with a positive outlook. Have this person say, "You... (And then the rest of the affirmation)."

After the 30 days, you will feel more confident, and your reservations about speaking into the voice recorder will diminish. Whatever remaining self-doubt or self-consciousness you have toward your voice, let it go. As you use your words, you start to experience even more profoundly positive changes to your self-confidence. During this time you can begin to use the important word, "I am."

Whenever you feel ready to move on, you can get rid of the recorder because it is time to use your newly developed positive mindset to speak to yourself.

Remember, we need to choose the right words to say to ourselves, so we don't self-sabotage. For instance, we don't want to say "I am no longer fat" we would want to say "I am skinny." Anytime we speak of a negative word we continue to breathe life into and it perpetuates.

As mentioned earlier there are various affirmations you can choose from which include:

1. **Affirm what you want to have."**
   "I am slim and toned."
   "I am muscular and thin."
   "I weight (x), it's my ideal weight."

2. **Affirm what you currently love about yourself.**
   "I love how dedicated I am to losing weight."
   "I love how good I feel after working out."
   "I love how I am finally taking time for myself."

3. **Affirm you are in control.**
   "I decide when I workout."
   "I choose to be happy."
   "I choose to eat healthy foods."

4. **Affirm that you know.**

"I know I will weigh (x) by (date)"

"I know that my body is getting stronger every day."

"I know my body is getting leaner every day."

5. **Affirm that you are grateful.**

"I am so happy and grateful for my body."

"I am so happy and grateful for delicious, healthy food."

"I am so happy and grateful for my workout time."

Keep in mind we are only using one affirmation for the first ten days. Deciding which one to use depends on what resonates best with you. For our clients we have them start by choosing one that speaks to how they "are in control."

We use these words because many of us we feel our lives are out of hand and that we don't have a decision in matters that affect us. By telling ourselves, "I am in control," or "I decide," we take the first step toward self –empowerment. This affirmation creates the momentum and grounding we need to move forward. If we are having another person speak the affirmation, have that person say,

"You are (the affirmation)" slowly and confidently for one minute.

During days 11-20 we have our clients "affirm what they want to have" and act as if they have it now. Once the foundation of declaring that you are in control is known, you can move onto what you really want. We act as if we have achieved this fitness or mental goal now because it gives us the motivation to continue to strive for it, for some this is known as the law of attraction.

Begin to think of what you want. It could be an ideal weight, having a toned body, whatever it might be, use this affirmation. Have the person say, "You are (x), and you have (y)." Again make sure they are saying these words slowly and confidently, this time for two minutes.

On the final stretch of days 21-30, we are now speaking three affirmations for a total of three minutes. During this phase we have our clients use the words: "I love..."

Now, if we had used the, "I love..." during the first 20 days, they would not have the same effect they now do on day 21.

By the 21st day, you have made the shift and have begun to change the neurological connections of your brain. When you listen to someone else say, "You love your (z)" profound changes happen.

Because they say you love (z), your brain will then say something like, "I do love my (z)."

Now on your 21st day, have that person in your life now use the power of all three affirmations for three minutes. Have them say, "You are (x) you have (y), and you love (z)." After hearing these for three minutes, you will feel so good about yourself you might even cry.

We've seen this happen many times before.

Because your mind is finally not rejecting affirmations, you begin to finally believe in their power. You then feel even more confident and self-assured than ever before.

As the week's progress, you can start to combine four affirmations and then five. We don't recommend any more than five affirmations because we've found it can scatter our focus. However, when you do reach the ability to listen to five affirmations and truly embody them, the sky is then the limit on how confident you will FEEL.

FINAL THOUGHTS

We hope you take the necessary steps we discussed and move closer each day to looking and feeling your best. Taking action is imperative to change because too many times we get stuck in our heads and never do anything to change. You must put what you have learned about into practice.

Don't just think about it, don't just talk about it and don't just read this book once.

You might be thinking, "You want me to read it again?"

Yes, we do!

There might be a little voice going in your head, screaming, "You are going to make me read this book again!"

Keep in mind repetition is the key to learning.

We experimented, tested and learned our way to success and now we want to pass on everything we know to you.

We want you to have a healthy and in shape body.

We want you to feel good about yourself and say nice things to yourself.

We want you to look in a mirror with a full sense of confidence.

We want you to look and feel your best.

You can do it,

We don't just believe it; we know you can do it!

WANT EVEN MORE?

Get ready to experience the Mind-Body Melt in Action....

Be sure to visit our YouTube Channel:

The Mind-Body Melt

There, you will find free sample workouts as well as meditations and affirmations which are specially designed to help you look and feel your best.

BUT... if you want to really want to reach your full potential, check out our website: www.TheMind-BodyMelt.com.

Here you will find our BREAKTHROUGH six-week holistic, *Mind-Body Melt Program* which takes you through 18 exercise routines, each specifically designed to help you to lose weight as well as look and feel your best. They come complete with meditations and affirmations at the end.

It comes in at the low cost of $97!

If you wanted to train 18 times with us that would cost over $2000!

Be sure to take advantage of this inexpensive opportunity before it's too late!

WHAT ARE YOU WAITING FOR?
TAKE ACTION RIGHT NOW!

ENDNOTES

1:
Rosenkilde, M., Auerbach, P., Reichkendler, M. H., Ploug, T., Stallknecht, B. M., & Sjödin, A. (2012, September 15). Body fat loss and compensatory mechanisms in response to different doses of aerobic exercise—a randomized controlled trial in overweight sedentary males. *American Journal of Physiology - Regulatory, Integrative and Comparative Physiology, 303*, 6th ser., R571-R579. doi:10.1152/ajpregu.00141.2012

2:
WHO | Physical Activity and Adults. (2016.). Retrieved October 17, 2016, from http://www.who.int/dietphysicalactivity/factsheet_adults/en/

3: Skoluda, N., et al., Elevated hair cortisol concentrations in endurance athletes. Psychoneuroendocrinology (2011), doi:10.1016/j.psyneuen.2011.09.001

4:

Target Heart Rate and Estimated Maximum Heart Rate. (2015, August 10). Retrieved October 17, 2016, from http://www.cdc.gov/physicalactivity/basics/measuring/heartrate.htm

5:

Roy, B. A. (2013). High-Intensity Interval Training. *ACSM's Health & Fitness Journal, 17*(3), 3. doi:10.1249/fit.0b013e31828cb21c

6:

Schuenke MD, Mikat RP, McBride JM (March 2002). "Effect of an acute period of resistance exercise on excess post-exercise oxygen consumption: implications for body mass management." European Journal of Applied Physiology. 86 (5): 411–7. doi:10.1007/s00421-001-0568-y. PMID 11882927

7:

Laforgia, J., Withers, R. T., & Gore, C. J. (2006). Effects of exercise intensity and duration on the excess post-exercise oxygen consumption. *Journal of Sports Sciences, 24*(12), 1247–1264. doi:10.1080/02640410600552064

8:

Slavin, J. L., & Lloyd, B. (2012). Health benefits of fruits and vegetables. *Advances in Nutrition: An International Review Journal, 3*(4), 506–516. doi:10.3945/an.112.002154

9:

Daniels, M. C., & Popkin, B. M. (2010, September). Impact of water intake on energy intake and weight status: A systematic review. Nutrv Rev., 9, 68-69. doi:10.1111/j.1753-4887.2010.00311.x.

10:

Stookey, J. D., Constant, F., Popkin, B. M., & Gardner, C. D. (2008). Drinking water is associated with weight loss in overweight dieting women independent of diet and activity. *Obesity, 16*(11), 2481–2488. doi:10.1038/oby.2008.409

11:

Davy, B. M., Dennis, E. A., Dengo, A. L., Wilson, K. L., & Davy, K. P. (2008). Water consumption reduces energy intake at a breakfast meal in obese older adults. *Journal of the American Dietetic Association, 108*(7), 1236–1239. doi:10.1016/j.jada.2008.04.013

12:

Brown, C. M., Dulloo, A. G., & Montani, J.-P. (2006). Water-induced Thermogenesis reconsidered: The effects of Osmolality and water temperature on energy expenditure after drinking. *The Journal of Clinical Endocrinology & Metabolism, 91*(9), 3598–3602. doi:10.1210/jc.2006-0407

13:Popkin, B. M., Barclay, D. V., & Nielsen, S. J. (2005). Water and food consumption patterns of U.S. Adults from 1999 to 2001. *Obesity Research, 13*(12), 2146–2152. doi:10.1038/oby.2005.266

14:

Ac, N. C. L. (2015, June). Learn how to unlock tissue memory. Retrieved October 17, 2016, from http://www.integrativehealthcare.org/mt/archives/2007/04/understanding_a.html

15:

Giovanni. (2015, January 7). 76 scientific benefits of meditation. Retrieved October 17, 2016, from meditation, http://liveanddare.com/benefits-of-meditation/

16:

McCorry, L. K. (2007). Physiology of the autonomic nervous system. *American Journal of Pharmaceutical Education, 71*(4), 78. doi:10.5688/aj710478

17:

Lee, A., & Campbell, D. (2009). *Perfect breathing: Transform your life, one breath at a time.* New York: Sterling Publishing.

18:

Publications, H. H. (2016, September 12). Relaxation techniques: Breath control helps quell errant stress response - Harvard health. Retrieved October 17, 2016, from http://www.health.harvard.edu/mind-and-mood/relaxation-techniques-breath-control-helps-quell-errant-stress-response

19:

Willis, J. (2008). *Teaching the brain to read: Strategies for improving fluency, vocabulary, and comprehension*. Alexandria, VA: Association for Supervision and Curriculum Development

20:

Goodenough, T. (2012, May 11). Vain or just paranoid? Women check their reflection EIGHT TIMES a day. *Daily Mail*. Retrieved from http://www.dailymail.co.uk/news/article-2142879/Looking-good-Women-check-reflection-times-day.html?ITO=1490

21:

Sims, L. (2012). *The workplace terrorist: A passport to keep you from becoming a workplace hostage. Take the Sims' flight*. United States: Iuniverse Com.

CPSIA information can be obtained
at www.ICGtesting.com
Printed in the USA
BVHW04s1934060618
518408BV00001B/104/P

9 780998 288307